AYURVEDA

COOKBOOK FOR WOMEN 2024

Harnessing the Healing Properties of Foods for Vitality, Hormone Balancing and Total Wellness

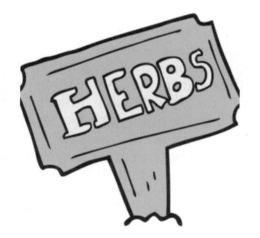

Manju Bhatti

Table of Contents

Introduction

"When diet is wrong, medicine is of no use. When diet is correct, medicine is of no need."

This ancient Ayurvedic saying eloquently conveys the profound wisdom that diet serves as more than just sustenance - it acts as a potent form of medicine that has the ability to rebalance our health and vitality. This is especially crucial for women, who experience a complex interplay of hormones throughout their lives, making the nourishing and healing power of food particularly impactful.

From the onset of menstruation to the journey through menopause, women undergo unique physiological shifts that require specific care. However, in today's fast-paced lifestyle, women often struggle to align with their natural rhythms, facing issues such as hormonal imbalances, irregular periods, mood fluctuations, and other health challenges. The encouraging truth is that Ayurveda, an ancient healing system from India, presents a holistic approach to women's well-being, highlighting the interconnectedness of body, mind, and spirit.

Ayurveda views each individual as a unique blend of three fundamental energies, or doshas: Vata, Pitta, and Kapha. These doshas govern both physical and mental functions, with their balance significantly influencing our health. Women typically exhibit a dominance of Vata and Pitta doshas, resulting in traits like creativity, sensitivity, and warmth, as well as

tendencies towards anxiety, stress, and hormonal imbalances.

Central to Ayurveda is the recognition that women's health is intricately linked to the cyclical patterns of the moon and the natural world. Menstruation, pregnancy, childbirth, and menopause are all phases that demand specific nourishment and care. Nevertheless, modern habits such as consuming processed foods, irregular sleep routines, and chronic stress often disturb these subtle rhythms, giving rise to various health issues

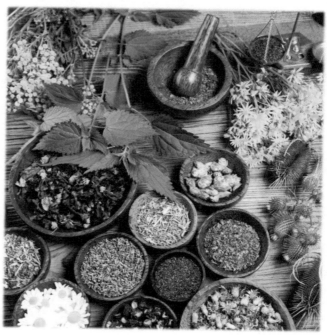

The Ayurvedic approach to women's health focuses on addressing the root cause of ailments rather than just alleviating symptoms. This entails understanding your unique constitution (Prakriti) and pinpointing any dosha imbalances (Vikriti) that may underlie your symptoms. Once you grasp your individual requirements, you can implement targeted dietary and lifestyle adjustments to bolster your body's innate healing capacities.

Diet plays a pivotal role in Ayurvedic practices, allowing you to create internal harmony by selecting foods that align with your dosha constitution and current phase of the menstrual cycle. This approach fosters hormonal equilibrium, diminishes inflammation, and enhances overall health. For instance, individuals with a Vata imbalance might find grounding and nourishing benefits in warm, cooked foods, whereas those with a Pitta imbalance may require cooling and soothing foods to pacify excess heat.

In addition to diet, Ayurveda presents a plethora of techniques for women's well-being, including herbal remedies, yoga, meditation, and massage. By integrating these practices into your daily life, you can further nurture your body's natural healing mechanisms and cultivate a profound sense of wellness.

Chapter 1

Ayurveda, known as the "Science of Life," is an ancient healing tradition that originated in India over 5,000 years ago. It offers a holistic approach to wellness, recognizing the intricate connection between the mind, body, and spirit. Emphasizing the significance of achieving internal and external balance, Ayurveda guides individuals towards a healthy and satisfying life.

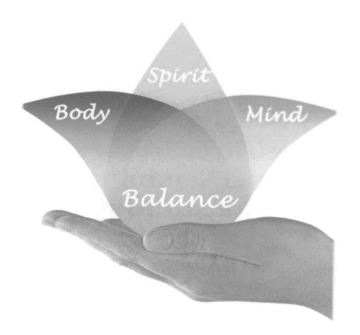

What is Ayurveda?

Ayurveda transcends being just a medical system; it embodies a way of life. The term is a combination of two Sanskrit words: "Ayu," meaning life, and "Veda," meaning knowledge or science, thus signifying "the knowledge of life." This comprehensive system encompasses various facets of health, including diet, lifestyle, herbal remedies, detoxification practices, yoga, meditation, and even astrology.

At its essence, Ayurveda centers on maintaining equilibrium among the three doshas, which are fundamental energies or biological humors present in each person. Vata, Pitta, and Kapha, derived from the elements ether (space), air, fire, water, and earth, govern different physiological and psychological functions. The unique blend of these doshas in an individual determines their constitution or "Prakriti."

Ayurveda and Women's Health

Ayurveda offers profound insights into women's health, acknowledging the distinct phases and transitions that occur throughout a woman's life. From menarche to menopause, each stage brings specific physiological and emotional changes, with Ayurveda providing tailored guidance to navigate these transitions gracefully.

Menstrual Cycle: Ayurveda views the menstrual cycle as a natural and vital cleansing process for the body. It offers specific dietary and lifestyle recommendations for each phase to enhance healthy flow, alleviate discomfort, and balance hormones.

Fertility and Pregnancy: Ayurveda embraces a holistic approach to enhance fertility and support a healthy pregnancy. This approach involves dietary modifications, herbal treatments, and lifestyle practices aimed at nurturing the well-being of both mother and baby.

Postpartum Care: Ayurvedic postpartum care underscores the importance of rest, rejuvenation, and nourishment for the new mother. Specific therapies like herbal baths and massages are recommended to facilitate recovery and encourage lactation.

Menopause: In Ayurveda, menopause is viewed as a natural life phase rather than a malady. It provides guidance on managing symptoms such as hot flashes, mood swings, and sleep disturbances through dietary adjustments, herbs, and lifestyle changes.

Diet and Lifestyle in Ayurveda

Ayurveda places great emphasis on the role of diet and lifestyle in preserving health and preventing ailments. Our food choices, daily habits, and routines profoundly influence our well-being.

Eating for Your Dosha: Ayurvedic dietary guidelines are tailored to an individual's dosha constitution. For instance, Vata types are advised to favor warm, cooked foods and avoid raw vegetables, while Pitta types should focus on cooling foods and limit spicy and oily dishes. Kapha types benefit from light, dry, and warming foods.

Mindful Eating: Ayurveda stresses mindful eating, encouraging us to eat slowly, relish each bite, and heed our body's hunger and fullness signals.

Seasonal Eating: Aligning our diet with the natural rhythms of the seasons is a fundamental principle in Ayurveda. It involves consuming seasonal foods believed to provide the nutrients required to adapt to the changing environment.

Daily Routine: Establishing a consistent daily routine, known as "dinacharya," is vital for maintaining balance and well-being. This routine includes early rising, yoga or exercise, meditation, regular meals, and sufficient sleep.

Herbal Remedies: Ayurveda harnesses a wide range of herbs and herbal formulations to address various health issues. These remedies are often customized to an individual's dosha constitution and specific requirements.

Detoxification: Regular detox practices, such as panchakarma (a five-fold purification process), are recommended in Ayurveda to rid the body of toxins and restore equilibrium.

The Ayurvedic Approach to Health

Ayurveda adopts a proactive and personalized approach to well-being, aiming to detect and manage imbalances early to prevent their progression into diseases. This is achieved through a comprehensive assessment of an individual's dosha constitution, lifestyle, diet, and emotional well-being.

Ayurvedic practitioners utilize various diagnostic tools, including pulse reading, tongue analysis, and observation of physical traits. Based on this evaluation, they devise a personalized treatment plan involving dietary adjustment, herbal remedies, lifestyle modifications, and detox therapies.

Ayurveda encourages individuals to take an active role in their health journey, promoting empowerment and self-care. It teaches us to listen to our bodies, understand our unique constitution, and make choices that foster balance and vitality. By embracing Ayurvedic principles, we can cultivate a life of health, harmony, and fulfillment.

The Three Doshas and the Feminine Constitution

Ayurveda, the ancient Indian science of life, recognizes the profound connection between nature and human health and well-being.

In the intricate world of a woman's body, hormones play a symphony of change and vitality, from the blossoming of menarche to the graceful transition of menopause. These chemical messengers orchestrate a delicate dance that shapes a woman's physical, emotional, and spiritual health. Ayurveda offers a unique lens to understand and nurture the feminine essence.

In the realm of Ayurveda, every individual is a unique tapestry woven with threads of the five fundamental elements – ether, air, fire, water, and earth, which combine to form the three doshas, or bio-energies, known as Vata, Pitta, and Kapha.

Each dosha governs specific physiological and psychological functions, and their interplay determines an individual's constitution or Prakriti. While everyone possesses all three doshas, their unique proportion varies, leading to distinct physical and mental characteristics.

Women experience a dynamic interplay of doshas throughout their lives due to the cyclical nature of their bodies. Hormonal fluctuations, menstrual cycles, pregnancy, childbirth, and menopause all influence the doshic balance, creating a need for personalized nourishment and care.

VATA

The Energy of Movement and Change

Vata, composed of ether and air, is the principle of movement and change, governing all bodily motions. Vata energy is often described as quick, lively, and enthusiastic, with a tendency towards spontaneity and change, especially prominent during menstruation and menopause.

When Vata is balanced, women experience regular menstrual cycles, healthy ovulation, and a vibrant libido, along with stable moods and mental clarity.

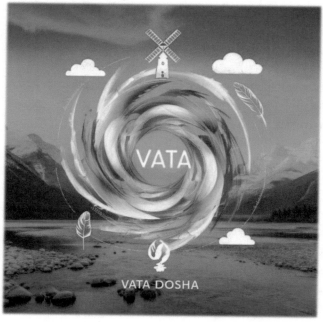

Vata Imbalance in Women

Symptoms of Vata imbalance in women may include irregular or painful periods, dry skin and hair, constipation, anxiety and insomnia, cold hands and feet, joint pain, and difficulty conceiving. To pacify Vata, women can incorporate grounding and warming practices into their daily routines, such as nourishing

foods like cooked vegetables, soups, stews, and warm milk, along with gentle exercises like yoga, tai chi, or walking to calm the nervous system.

PITTA

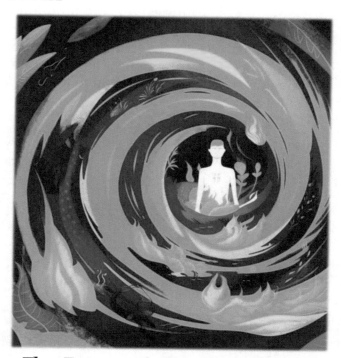

The Energy of Transformation and Metabolism

Pitta, composed of fire and water, is the principle of transformation and metabolism, governing digestion and nutrient assimilation. Pitta energy is described as sharp, focused, and determined, often heightened during ovulation and the premenstrual phase.

When Pitta is balanced, women experience regular menstrual flow, healthy ovulation, strong digestion, radiant skin, and a sharp intellect, along with balanced emotions and confidence.

Pitta Imbalance in Women

Imbalance in Pitta may lead to skin issues, heartburn, excessive thirst, irritability, anger, and heavy bleeding during menstruation. To restore balance, the Pitta woman should focus on cooling practices, including a diet rich in fresh fruits, vegetables, and cooling herbs, while avoiding spicy and oily foods. Moderate exercise, cooling pranayama practices, time in nature, and herbal remedies can also support hormonal balance and reduce inflammation.

KAPHA
The Energy of Structure and Stability

Kapha, composed of earth and water, provides structure, lubrication, and immunity, essential for maintaining healthy tissues in women. Balanced Kapha results in regular menstrual cycles, strong bones, lustrous hair, and a calm mind, along with stable emotions and compassion.

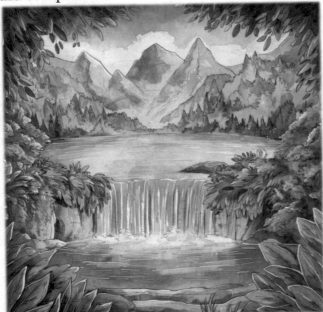

Kapha Imbalance in Women

Imbalance in Kapha may manifest as weight gain, sluggish digestion, congestion, lethargy, depression, and heavy periods. To restore balance, the Kapha woman should focus on stimulating practices, including a diet rich in light, warming foods and spices, along with regular exercise to increase metabolism and circulation. Invigorating activities, dry brushing, stimulating pranayama practices, and herbal remedies can also support digestion, metabolism, and hormonal balance.

Nourishing the Feminine Essence with Ayurveda

Ayurveda offers a holistic approach to women's health, recognizing the interconnectedness of mind, body, and spirit. By understanding their unique doshic constitution and embracing personalized practices, women can achieve optimal health.

Specific recommendations for women's health concerns, including recipes, herbal remedies, and lifestyle practices, aim to nourish the feminine essence and promote balance throughout life stages.

By aligning with Ayurvedic wisdom, women can unlock their healing potential and cultivate radiant health. Remember, Ayurveda is not one-size-fits-all. Listening to your body, observing its rhythms, and making choices that support your needs are key.

The Ayurvedic Approach to Hormonal Health

"The body of a woman is a temple, and her hormones are the sacred music that orchestrates its rhythms."

This ancient Ayurvedic saying beautifully expresses the deep connection between women's health and their hormonal balance. Hormones play a crucial role in influencing various aspects of life, including mood, energy levels, fertility, and overall well-being. However, in today's fast-paced world, many women struggle with hormonal imbalances, which can lead to discomfort and health issues.

Ayurveda, an ancient science of life, provides a holistic and individualized approach to comprehending and restoring hormonal harmony. Rooted in the principles of balance and interconnectedness, Ayurveda considers hormonal health as a vital component of women's overall well-being. By addressing the underlying causes of imbalances and nourishing the body with specific foods, herbs, and lifestyle practices, Ayurveda empowers women to regain their natural rhythms and achieve optimal health.

Understanding The Hormonal Dance

Hormones act as chemical messengers that travel throughout the body, regulating a wide range of physiological processes. In women, these messengers control functions such as the menstrual cycle, fertility, pregnancy, and menopause. Key hormones involved in this intricate process include estrogen, progesterone, testosterone, and thyroid hormones.

When hormones are in harmony, women experience regular menstrual cycles, healthy fertility, stable moods, and high energy levels. However, various factors can disrupt this delicate balance. Elements such as stress, poor diet, lack of sleep, environmental toxins, and certain medications can all contribute to hormonal imbalances.

Common signs of hormonal imbalances in women may include:

- Irregular menstrual cycles
- Mood swings and irritability
- Fatigue and low energy
- Difficulty sleeping
- Weight changes
- Hair loss or thinning
- Skin issues like acne
- Decreased libido
- Difficulty conceiving

Ayurveda's Unique Perspective

Ayurveda considers hormonal imbalances as reflections of imbalances in the body's three doshas – Vata, Pitta, and Kapha. These doshas represent the fundamental energies that govern all physiological and psychological processes.

Vata dosha, associated with air and space, governs movement and communication within the body. An imbalance in Vata can lead to symptoms such as irregular menstrual cycles, anxiety, insomnia, and dryness.

Pitta dosha, linked to fire and water, oversees metabolism and transformation. When Pitta is imbalanced, it can result in issues like heavy menstrual flow, hot flashes, irritability, and inflammation.

Kapha dosha, related to earth and water, is in charge of stability and structure. An imbalance in Kapha may manifest as weight gain, lethargy, low mood, and fertility challenges.

Ayurveda recognizes that each woman has a unique constitution, or Prakriti, which is determined by the predominance of these doshas. This constitution forms the basis of her health and well-being. Optimal health is experienced when the doshas are balanced, but if one or more doshas become aggravated, it can lead to hormonal imbalances and other health issues.

Restoring Balance Through Ayurveda

Ayurveda offers a comprehensive and personalized approach to balancing hormones, involving:

Identifying the Root Cause: Ayurvedic practitioners conduct a detailed assessment of a woman's Prakriti, current health status, and lifestyle to pinpoint the root cause of her hormonal imbalance. This assessment may include pulse diagnosis, tongue analysis, and a thorough questionnaire about diet, sleep habits, stress levels, and other relevant factors.

Personalized Diet and Lifestyle Recommendations: Based on the assessment, Ayurvedic practitioners develop a customized plan that includes dietary guidelines, lifestyle adjustments, herbal remedies, and other therapeutic approaches.

Diet: Ayurveda highlights the importance of consuming a diet that aligns with one's individual constitution and the current season. This may involve incorporating specific tastes and qualities of food to balance the aggravated dosha. For example, a woman with a Vata imbalance might be advised to eat warm, cooked foods that are grounding and nourishing, while a woman with a Pitta imbalance may be recommended to favor cooling foods and avoid spicy or oily dishes.

Lifestyle: Ayurvedic practitioners also suggest lifestyle modifications that promote hormonal balance, such as establishing a consistent sleep routine, practicing stress-relief techniques like yoga and meditation, and engaging in gentle exercise.

Herbal Remedies: Ayurveda offers a vast array of herbs to support hormonal health, which can be consumed as teas, powders, capsules, or tinctures. Some common Ayurvedic herbs for women's health include Shatavari, Ashwagandha, Guduchi, and Ashoka.

Other Therapeutic Modalities: In addition to diet, lifestyle, and herbs, Ayurvedic practitioners may recommend various therapeutic modalities like Panchakarma (a detoxification and rejuvenation therapy), Abhyanga (Ayurvedic oil massage), and Shirodhara (a technique involving warm oil poured over the forehead).

The Ayurvedic Diet

In Ayurveda, food serves as more than just sustenance; it is considered medicine. A balanced Ayurvedic diet not only nourishes the body and supports hormonal function but also promotes overall well-being. Key principles of an Ayurvedic diet for hormonal health include:

Prioritizing Whole, Unprocessed Foods: Opt for fresh, seasonal fruits and vegetables, whole grains, legumes, nuts, and seeds while minimizing processed foods, refined sugars, and unhealthy fats.

Eating According to Your Dosha: Tailor your diet to your dosha type – Vata types benefit from warm, cooked foods and healthy fats, Pitta types thrive on cooling foods like cucumbers and leafy greens, and Kapha types do well with light, dry foods and spices.

Incorporating Hormone-Balancing Foods: Include specific foods known for their properties that support hormonal health, such as:

Shatavari: A revered herb that helps nourish and balance female hormones.

Ashwagandha: An adaptogenic herb that aids in stress management and supports healthy adrenal function.

Sesame Seeds: Rich in lignans, which are phytoestrogens that can assist in regulating estrogen levels.

Flaxseeds: Another source of lignans, as well as omega-3 fatty acids crucial for hormone production.

Leafy Greens: Packed with essential vitamins and minerals for hormonal health.

Cruciferous Vegetables: Contain compounds that promote healthy estrogen metabolism.

By embracing an Ayurvedic diet, you provide your body with the necessary nutrients and energy to maintain hormonal balance and thrive.

Lifestyle Practices

In Ayurveda, a balanced lifestyle is deemed just as important as a healthy diet. Key lifestyle practices for hormonal health include:

Regular Exercise: Engage in moderate physical activities like yoga, walking, or swimming to help regulate hormones, reduce stress, and enhance overall well-being.

Stress Management: Chronic stress can significantly impact your hormones. Find healthy stress management techniques such as meditation, deep breathing exercises, or spending time in nature.

Adequate Sleep: Make quality sleep a priority and aim for 7-8 hours of rest each night as it is essential for hormone regulation and overall health.

Mindful Eating: Practice mindful eating by savoring each bite, fully focusing on the flavors of your food, and stopping when you feel comfortably full. Avoid distractions such as watching TV or working while eating.

Daily Routine: Establish a consistent daily schedule that includes regular meal times and a bedtime routine. This consistency helps regulate your body's natural rhythms and promotes hormonal balance.

Women's Health Throughout the Life Cycle

Ayurveda, the ancient Indian system of medicine, offers a holistic approach to women's health that respects the natural rhythms and transitions experienced throughout the female life cycle. From menarche to motherhood and menopause, Ayurveda provides insights and practices to support each stage. By recognizing the unique requirements of each phase, women can harness the power of Ayurveda to optimize their health, well-being, and vitality.

Menarche

Menarche, the first occurrence of menstruation, signifies a significant milestone in a young woman's life, marking the transition from childhood to adolescence and the awakening of her reproductive potential. During this period, it is crucial to establish healthy habits that support hormonal balance and overall well-being.

According to Ayurveda, menarche is characterized as a Vata-dominant phase, exhibiting qualities of dryness, lightness, and coldness.To counter these qualities, young women should focus on a warming, grounding diet comprising cooked foods, healthy fats, and warming spices such as ginger and cinnamon. Regular meals and sufficient sleep are also vital to maintain energy levels and prevent Vata aggravation.

Ayurvedic Practices for Menarche

Nourishing Diet: Include warm, cooked foods like soups, stews, and grains. Favor sweet, sour, and salty tastes while avoiding excessive raw, cold, or dry foods.

Herbal Support: Consider incorporating herbal teas or supplements like Shatavari, known for its hormone-balancing properties.

Warm Oil Massage (Abhyanga): Regularly massage the body with warm sesame oil to pacify Vata and induce relaxation.

Gentle Exercise: Engage in moderate activities like yoga or walking to support circulation and reduce stress.

Rest and Relaxation: Prioritize adequate sleep and rest to replenish energy levels and balance hormones.

Motherhood

Motherhood encompasses pregnancy, childbirth, and postpartum recovery, representing a profound and transformative journey for women. Ayurveda offers valuable guidance during this sacred period, emphasizing the significance of nourishment, rest, and emotional support.

Pregnancy

During pregnancy, Ayurveda recommends a nutrient-rich diet to support both the growing baby and the mother's health. Essential components include warm, cooked foods, ghee (clarified butter), and easily digestible proteins. Certain herbs and foods such as raw, cold, and processed foods should be avoided during pregnancy for safety reasons.

Postpartum

Postpartum care focuses on restoring the mother's energy levels and supporting lactation. Recommendations include consuming warm, nourishing foods like soups, stews, and herbal teas, along with gentle massage and adequate rest.

Ayurvedic Practices for Motherhood

Pregnancy Diet: Emphasize warm, cooked foods, ghee, and easily digestible proteins while avoiding raw, cold, and processed foods.

Postpartum Diet: Continue with warm, nourishing foods and incorporate galactagogues such as fennel, cumin, and fenugreek to promote lactation.

Herbal Support: Consult an Ayurvedic practitioner for personalized herbal recommendations during pregnancy and the postpartum period.

Rest and Relaxation: Prioritize rest and sleep to aid recovery and replenish energy levels.

Gentle Exercise: Engage in light exercises like walking or gentle yoga once the initial postpartum period has passed.

Menopause

Menopause signals the conclusion of a woman's reproductive years and can bring about various physical and emotional changes due to declining estrogen levels. Ayurveda views menopause as another Vata-dominant phase, similar to menarche. Symptoms such as hot flashes, night sweats, and mood swings can be experienced during this time.

Ayurveda offers a holistic approach to managing menopausal symptoms by pacifying Vata dosha and promoting hormonal balance. Through a nourishing diet, herbal remedies, and lifestyle adjustments, discomfort can be alleviated, and overall well-being can be enhanced.

Ayurvedic Practices for Menopause

Cooling Diet: Opt for cooling foods like fruits, vegetables, and dairy products while avoiding spicy, fried, and processed foods.

Herbal Support: Consider incorporating herbs like Shatavari, Ashwagandha, and Brahmi to balance hormones and reduce stress.

Oil Massage (Abhyanga): Regular oil massages using cooling oils like coconut oil can help pacify Vata and alleviate hot flashes.

Gentle Exercise: Engage in regular physical activities like yoga, walking, or swimming to manage stress and support bone health.

Stress Management: Practice relaxation techniques such as meditation, deep breathing, and yoga Nidra to reduce stress levels and improve sleep quality.

Ayurvedic Principles

In addition to specific practices for each stage of life, Ayurveda emphasizes several general principles for women's health:

Balanced Diet: A balanced diet based on the six tastes (sweet, sour, salty, bitter, pungent, and astringent) is essential for overall health and well-being.

Regular Routine: Establishing a daily routine that includes adequate sleep, regular meals, and time for relaxation is crucial for hormonal balance and stress management.

Mindful Eating: Eating mindfully, without distractions, and paying attention to hunger and fullness cues can improve digestion and prevent overeating.

Herbal Support: Ayurvedic herbs and supplements can be used to address specific health concerns and promote overall well-being.

Lifestyle Practices: Yoga, meditation, and pranayama (breathing exercises) can help reduce stress, improve sleep, and enhance overall health.

Creating a Personalized Ayurvedic Routine for Women

Ayurveda, the ancient Indian system of medicine, offers a holistic approach to health and well-being, recognizing the interconnectedness of mind, body, and spirit. A cornerstone of Ayurvedic practice is the understanding that each individual possesses a unique constitution, or "Prakriti," determined by the balance of three fundamental energies known as doshas: Vata, Pitta, and Kapha.

Women, in particular, experience a dynamic interplay of these doshas throughout their lives, influenced by hormonal fluctuations, menstrual cycles, pregnancy, and menopause. By recognizing your individual constitution and understanding how it interacts with the rhythms of your body, you can create a personalized Ayurvedic routine that supports hormonal balance, enhances well-being, and empowers you to live in harmony with your natural cycles.

Understanding Your Dosha, The Key to Personalization

In Ayurveda, each dosha is associated with specific physical, emotional, and mental characteristics.

Vata: Characterized by qualities of movement, lightness, and dryness. Vata-dominant women tend to be creative, energetic, and quick-witted but may also experience anxiety, irregular digestion, and dry skin.

Pitta: Associated with qualities of heat, transformation, and intensity. Pitta-dominant women often possess a strong intellect, leadership qualities, and a radiant complexion but may also be prone to inflammation, skin irritations, and a quick temper.

Kapha: Represents qualities of stability, grounding, and nourishment. Kapha-dominant women are typically calm, compassionate, and nurturing but may also struggle with weight gain, sluggishness, and congestion.

While most individuals possess a combination of all three doshas, one or two typically predominate, shaping their overall constitution. By understanding your dominant dosha(s), you can tailor your diet, lifestyle, and self-care practices to maintain balance and promote optimal health.

Crafting Your Personalized Ayurvedic Routine

Once you have a good understanding of your dosha, you can begin to create a daily routine that supports your unique needs. Here are some key areas to consider:

Diet

Vata: Favor warm, cooked foods that are grounding and nourishing. Incorporate healthy fats, such as ghee and coconut oil, and warming spices like ginger and cinnamon. Avoid cold, raw foods and caffeine, which can aggravate Vata.

Pitta: Opt for cooling and hydrating foods, such as cucumber, coconut, and sweet fruits. Limit spicy, fried, and sour foods, which can increase Pitta.

Kapha: Choose light, dry, and warming foods. Incorporate plenty of vegetables, legumes, and whole grains. Avoid heavy, oily, and sweet foods, which can exacerbate Kapha.

Lifestyle

Vata: Establish a consistent routine with regular mealtimes and sleep schedules. Engage in calming activities, such as gentle yoga, meditation, and spending time in nature. Avoid overstimulation and excessive activity.

Pitta: Prioritize activities that promote relaxation and cooling, such as swimming, walking in nature, and restorative yoga. Avoid excessive heat and competition.

Kapha: Incorporate invigorating activities, such as brisk walking, jogging, and dancing. Challenge yourself with new experiences and avoid excessive sleep and sedentary behavior.

Self-Care

Vata: Regularly practice self-massage with warm sesame oil to soothe the nervous system and promote relaxation. Incorporate grounding and calming aromatherapy, such as lavender and chamomile.

Pitta: Use cooling and soothing skincare products, such as aloe vera and rosewater. Practice calming breathing exercises and prioritize relaxation.

Kapha: Engage in stimulating self-massage with warming oils, such as mustard or olive oil. Incorporate invigorating aromatherapy, such as peppermint and eucalyptus.

Herbal Support

Vata: Ashwagandha, Shatavari, and licorice root can help balance Vata.

Pitta: Brahmi, Amalaki, and Neem can help pacify Pitta.

Kapha: Triphala, Turmeric, and Ginger can help reduce Kapha.

Honoring Your Menstrual Cycle

For women, the menstrual cycle is a powerful rhythm that influences both physical and emotional well-being. Ayurveda provides specific guidance for each phase of the cycle, emphasizing the importance of adjusting diet, lifestyle, and self-care practices to support the body's natural processes.

Menstrual Phase: During menstruation, focus on rest, relaxation, and nourishment. Favor warm, cooked foods, such as soups and stews, and avoid strenuous activity. Incorporate gentle yoga poses and calming herbs like chamomile and lavender.

Follicular Phase: As energy levels rise, gradually increase activity and incorporate more fresh fruits and vegetables into your diet. This is a great time for creative projects and social activities.

Ovulatory Phase: Embrace your peak energy levels and focus on nourishing your body with a balanced diet. Continue to incorporate movement and exercise into your routine.

Luteal Phase: As the body prepares for menstruation, prioritize rest and relaxation. Favor warm, comforting foods and avoid stimulants like caffeine and alcohol. Engage in calming practices, such as meditation and gentle yoga.

Embracing Change and Adapting Your Routine

It's important to remember that your dosha constitution and needs may shift over time, influenced by factors such as stress, diet, and lifestyle changes. Be attentive to your body's signals and adjust your routine accordingly.

By embracing the principles of Ayurveda and tailoring your daily practices to your unique constitution, you can create a personalized routine that supports hormonal balance, enhances well-being, and empowers you to live in harmony with your natural rhythms.

Additional Tips for Creating Your Personalized Ayurvedic Routine:

Consult an Ayurvedic practitioner: A qualified practitioner can provide personalized guidance and recommendations based on your individual constitution and health concerns.

Keep a journal: Track your daily habits, energy levels, and any physical or emotional changes you experience. This can help you identify patterns and make adjustments to your routine as needed.

Be patient: It takes time to establish a new routine and see results. Be kind to yourself and trust the process.

Listen to your body: Your body is your greatest teacher. Pay attention to how you feel after eating certain foods, engaging in specific activities, or using different self-care practices.

Experiment: Ayurveda is not a one-size-fits-all approach. Don't be afraid to experiment with different practices and find what works best for you.

Chapter 2

The Six Tastes and Their Balancing Effects

Ayurveda, an ancient Indian science, views food as more than just fuel for our bodies; it's also medicine. Every bite we take has a unique energy that affects our health and well-being. Understanding this connection between food and health is key in Ayurveda. A central concept in this practice is the six tastes, which guide how we cook and eat.

The Six Tastes (Shad Rasa)

Ayurveda recognizes six tastes, each made up of two of the five elements: ether, air, fire, water, and earth. Here's a simple breakdown:

Sweet (Madhura): Earth + Water
- What It Does: Sweet taste is comforting and nourishing. It's cooling and helps build strength and vitality.
- Examples: Fruits, grains, dairy, honey, jaggery.
- Too Much: Can cause weight gain, sluggishness, and high blood sugar.

Sour (Amla): Earth + Fire
- What It Does: Sour taste stimulates digestion and awakens the appetite. It helps absorb nutrients and supports gut health.
- Examples: Citrus fruits, yogurt, sauerkraut, vinegar.
- Too Much: Can cause acidity, heartburn, and inflammation.

Salty (Lavana): Water + Fire
- What It Does: Salty taste is grounding and hydrating. It supports digestion and maintains electrolyte balance.
- Examples: Sea salt, Himalayan pink salt.
- Too Much: Can lead to water retention, high blood pressure, and kidney problems.

Pungent (Katu): Fire + Air
- What It Does: Pungent taste is warming and stimulates circulation. It boosts metabolism and helps with weight loss.
- Examples: Chili peppers, ginger, garlic, onions, black pepper.
- Too Much: Can irritate the digestive system and cause inflammation.

Bitter (Tikta): Air + Ether
- What It Does: Bitter taste is cooling and detoxifying. It stimulates the liver and aids digestion.
- Examples: Leafy greens, cruciferous vegetables, turmeric, neem.
- Too Much: Can lead to dryness and depletion.

Astringent (Kashaya): Air + Earth
- What It Does: Astringent taste is cooling and drying. It reduces inflammation and tightens tissues.
- Examples: Legumes, pomegranate, cranberries, unripe bananas.
- Too Much: Can cause constipation and dryness.

Balancing the Tastes for Optimal Health

Ayurveda suggests that a healthy diet includes all six tastes in moderation. Each taste affects the doshas (body energies) differently, so understanding these effects helps you tailor your diet to your unique needs.

Vata Constitution: If you often feel dry, cold, and light, you might need more sweet, sour, and salty tastes to feel grounded and nourished.

Pitta Constitution: If you tend to be hot, intense, and sharp, focusing on bitter, sweet, and astringent tastes can help cool and balance you.

Kapha Constitution: If you often feel heavy, slow, and cold, incorporating more pungent, bitter, and astringent tastes can stimulate your metabolism and reduce stagnation.

Since everyone is different, the right balance of tastes varies from person to person. It's best to consult with an Ayurvedic practitioner to create a personalized diet plan.

The Art of Ayurvedic Cooking

Ayurvedic cooking combines different tastes and ingredients to make meals that are balanced and nourishing. It uses fresh, seasonal ingredients and spices to enhance the healing properties of food.

Including all six tastes in your meals is easy. You can start with a variety of vegetables, fruits, grains, legumes, and healthy fats. Use spices and herbs to add flavor and therapeutic benefits.

Example of a Balanced Ayurvedic Meal:

- A sweet potato or squash dish (sweet)
- A leafy green salad with lemon vinaigrette (sour and bitter)
- A lentil soup or dal (salty and astringent)
- A vegetable stir-fry with ginger and garlic (pungent)

Ayurvedic Spices

Ayurveda recognizes spices' power to enhance flavor and promote healing. For women, spices offer benefits like hormonal health support, boosted energy, improved digestion, and enhanced beauty. Let's explore key Ayurvedic spices and their advantages for women.

Turmeric

Known for its golden hue, turmeric is essential in Ayurveda and Indian cuisine. Curcumin in turmeric has anti-inflammatory and antioxidant properties, alleviating menstrual cramps, regulating cycles, supporting hormonal balance, promoting skin health, aiding detoxification, and improving digestion. Add turmeric to curries, soups, smoothies, or enjoy golden milk before bed.

Ginger

Renowned for its warming and digestive properties, ginger ignites the digestive fire, improves circulation, alleviates nausea, reduces inflammation, and eases menstrual discomfort. Add fresh ginger to teas, stir-fries, or soups for wellness benefits.

Cumin

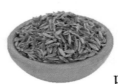

With an earthy aroma, cumin seeds aid digestion by stimulating digestive enzymes, reducing bloating, promoting bowel movements, and providing iron, important for women prone to iron deficiency. Use cumin in soups, vegetable dishes, or on roasted vegetables.

Coriander

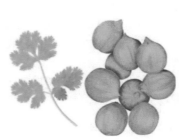

Coriander aids digestion, reduces inflammation, regulates blood sugar, and detoxifies, supporting liver and kidney functions. Use coriander seeds in cooking or add fresh cilantro leaves to salads, salsas, or soups.

Fennel

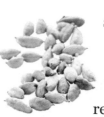

Fennel seeds, with a sweet flavor, ease menstrual cramps, support digestion, reduce bloating, and promote lactation. Enjoy fennel tea after meals or chew fennel seeds for fresh breath.

Cardamom

Cardamom pods, with a sweet aroma, act as aphrodisiacs, stimulate senses, improve circulation, support libido, aid digestion, and reduce water retention. Add cardamom to rice dishes, desserts, or teas.

Cinnamon

Popular for its warm flavor, cinnamon helps regulate blood sugar, provides anti-inflammatory and antioxidant benefits. Top oatmeal, yogurt, or baked goods with a dash of cinnamon.

Black Pepper

Black pepper enhances nutrient absorption, especially with turmeric, aids digestion, relieves gas, and promotes circulation.

Additional Ayurvedic Spices

Apart from the mentioned spices, others beneficial for women include:

- Fenugreek: Increases milk production, regulates blood sugar, aids weight management.
- Ajwain: Aids digestion, relieves gas, bloating, menstrual cramps.
- Asafoetida: Reduces bloating, aids digestion.
- Nutmeg: Supports digestion, relieves stress.
- Cloves: Help with toothaches, oral health, possess analgesic properties.

Important Herbs for Women's Health

In Ayurveda, an ancient healing system, there are some special herbs that have been loved for a long time for how they help women stay healthy. These herbs can be really good for things like keeping hormones balanced, making periods more comfortable, helping with getting pregnant, keeping emotions in check, and making menopause easier. Let's learn about some of these herbs and what they can do for women's bodies.

Shatavari

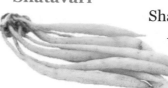

Shatavari is also called Asparagus racemosus and is known as the "queen of herbs" in Ayurveda because it's great for women's health. It helps the female reproductive system, keeps hormones balanced, supports getting pregnant, and eases period pains and menopause symptoms. Shatavari has plant compounds that are like estrogen, which is a female hormone. These compounds can help regulate periods, lessen PMS symptoms like mood swings, and even boost sex drive. Besides helping with hormones, Shatavari can also help new moms make more breast milk, support the immune system, aid digestion, and help with emotions.

Ashwagandha

Ashwagandha, scientifically known as Withania somnifera, is a top herb in Ayurveda known as an adaptogen. Adaptogens are natural things that help the body handle stress and stay balanced during tough times. For women, stress can mess up hormones and cause issues like irregular periods, mood swings, and trouble getting pregnant. Ashwagandha can help the body deal with stress, which can then keep hormones in check. Studies have found that Ashwagandha can lower a stress hormone called cortisol, and by doing this, it can indirectly help make other hormones that are important for regular periods and fertility. Ashwagandha can also help with anxiety, depression, thyroid health, energy levels, and brain function.

Guduchi

Guduchi, also known as Tinospora cordifolia, is a strong herb known for helping the immune system and purifying the blood. In Ayurveda, having a strong immune system is key to good health, and Guduchi is often recommended to help the body fight infections. For women, a good immune system is extra important during pregnancy and after giving birth when the body is going through many changes and is more likely to get sick. Guduchi can boost the production of white blood cells, which are important for fighting off germs. It also reduces inflammation, cleans the blood, and gets rid of toxins. This cleansing process can help with skin health, periods, and overall energy.

Manjistha

Manjistha, scientifically known as Rubia cordifolia, is a herb that cleans the blood and lymphatic system. The lymphatic system removes waste and toxins from the body, which is important for good health. For women, this system plays a role in hormones and skin health. Manjistha helps get rid of extra hormones and toxins in the blood, which can cause period problems, acne, and other skin issues. It also fights inflammation, good for skin conditions like eczema, and improves circulation for healthy and glowing skin.

Brahmi

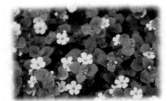

Brahmi, or Bacopa monnieri, is a famous herb for boosting the brain and reducing stress. In Ayurveda, it's known for enhancing memory, intelligence, and clear thinking. For women with lots to do, brahmi can help manage stress and keep the mind healthy. Brahmi can improve memory, learning, attention, and mood. It also reduces anxiety, helps with relaxation, and supports good sleep, which is important for health and hormones.

Ghee - The Magic Ayurvedic Ingredient

In the special kitchens of Ayurveda, where food and healing come together, ghee is like a magic potion. It's known for its special powers and seen as very important for life. Ghee is made by heating butter and has many benefits for women's health, helping them feel strong and healthy.

What is Ghee?

Ghee is not just like any other cooking oil - it is full of good things that help our bodies, gives us energy, and makes us feel good. In Ayurveda, ghee is thought to be a pure and balancing food that keeps our bodies and minds healthy.

Why is Ghee Good for You?

Ghee has butyric acid that keeps our stomach and intestines healthy, helping us digest food better and get rid of bad stuff in our bodies. It's also rich in vitamins that boost our immune system, keep our bones strong, and make our skin glow. Another good thing in ghee is CLA, which helps our bodies work better and burn fat.

How Ghee Helps Women

Ghee is extra helpful for women who want to keep their hormones in balance. Whether you want to have a regular period, get pregnant, have a healthy baby, or go through menopause more easily, ghee can help you feel better.

Staying Healthy with Ghee

You can use ghee in many ways to stay healthy every day:

- **Cooking:** Use ghee for cooking your food as it is really good for you and makes your meals tasty.
- **Herbal Mixtures:** Mix ghee with herbs to make natural remedies that help your body.
- **Skin Care:** Massage a little bit of warm ghee on your skin to keep it soft and relaxed.
- **Golden Milk:** Drink a warm cup of golden milk with ghee before bedtime for a good night's sleep.

Choosing the Best Ghee

When you buy ghee, choose organic and grass-fed ghee for the best quality. Make sure it is made from cultured butter, which is easier to digest, especially if you are sensitive to dairy.

A Quick Note

Even though ghee is healthy, remember to enjoy it in moderation as it is high in calories. If you are allergic to dairy, it's best to avoid ghee.

Ghee is a wonderful natural ingredient that keeps us healthy in body, mind, and spirit. By using ghee every day, you can feel stronger and live a healthy life.

Ayurvedic Cooking Methods

Cooking is not just about making food; it's about creating a strong bond with your food and your body. Ayurvedic cooking tips can help you change your kitchen into a place for keeping your hormones balanced and staying healthy.

Ayurveda sees cooking as a loving and respectful way of using ingredients. It's about valuing the natural energy (prana) of each food and keeping its life-giving properties. This careful way of cooking makes your meals tastier and healthier, and it also helps your body stay balanced and in harmony.

Keeping Food Fresh

Ayurveda prefers gentle cooking methods that retain the important energy of food, unlike regular cooking that often uses high heat. Here are some important Ayurvedic cooking ideas to use in your kitchen:

- **Steaming:** Keeps the nutrients and moisture in vegetables, grains, and legumes. Great for Vata dosha as it adds moisture and warmth.
- **Sautéing:** Quick cooking over medium heat with a bit of oil or ghee. Good for all doshas, especially balancing for Pitta because it's cooling.
- **Slow Cooking:** Lets flavors mix together over time, perfect for stews, soups, and dals. Very helpful for Vata dosha as it gives a sense of stability and warmth.
- **Baking:** A flexible method for many dishes, but use moderate heat to prevent overcooking.
- **Avoid Deep-Frying:** Not recommended in Ayurveda as it makes heavy foods that are hard to digest and can disturb all three doshas.

Mindful Preparation and Consumption

In Ayurveda, how you prepare and eat your food is as important as the ingredients. Here are some tips for mindful eating:

- **Cook with Love:** See cooking as a way to meditate, focusing on the present moment.
- **Eat Fresh:** Use fresh, seasonal, locally grown organic ingredients when possible.

- **Eat Mindfully:** Sit down to eat without distractions, chew your food properly, and enjoy each bite.
- **Listen to Your Body:** Notice when you're hungry or full, and stop eating when you're satisfied.
- **Give Thanks:** Be grateful for the nourishment your food gives you.

Ayurvedic Cooking for Women's Health

Ayurvedic cooking is great for supporting women's bodies and hormones. Here are some tips for women:

- Choose Warming and Grounding Foods: Balance Vata by eating warm cooked vegetables, soups, stews, and grains.
- Add Healthy Fats: Ghee, coconut oil, and avocado oil are important for hormonal health, so include them in your diet in small amounts.
- Go for Seasonal and Local Foods: Eating seasonal food helps your body stay healthy, so pick local produce when you can.
- Use Herbs and Spices Wisely: Herbs like shatavari, ashwagandha, and fennel are very good for women's health, so include them in your meals.
- Personalize Your Diet: Customize your diet based on your own body and any health issues you have. Talk to an Ayurvedic practitioner for a plan that fits your needs.

Basic Kitchen Measurements and Conversions

Liquid Ingredients

Unit	Equivalent
1 teaspoon (tsp)	4.93 milliliters (ml)
1 tablespoon (tbsp)	14.79 milliliters (ml)
1 fluid ounce (fl oz)	29.57 milliliters (ml)
1 cup	237 milliliters (ml)
1 pint (pt)	473 milliliters (ml)

Dry Ingredients

Unit	Equivalent
1 teaspoon (tsp)	4.93 milliliters (ml)
1 tablespoon (tbsp)	14.79 milliliters (ml)
1 ounce (oz)	28.35 grams (g)
1 cup flour	120 grams (g)
1 cup sugar	200 grams (g)

US to Metric

US Unit	Metric Equivalent
1 inch	2.54 centimeters (cm)
1 foot	30.48 centimeters (cm)
1 yard	0.91 meters (m)
1 mile	1.61 kilometers (km)
1 pound (lb)	0.45 kilograms (kg)

Weights

Unit	Equivalent
1 ounce (oz)	28.35 grams (g)
1 pound (lb)	453.59 grams (g)
1 kilogram (kg)	2.20 pounds (lbs)
1 stone (st)	6.35 kilograms (kg)
1 metric ton	1000 kilograms (kg)

Baking in Grams

Ingredient	US Unit	Grams (g)
All-purpose flour	1 cup	120 grams
Granulated sugar	1 cup	200 grams
Brown sugar	1 cup packed	220 grams
Butter	1 cup	227 grams
Rolled oats	1 cup	90 grams

Oven Temperature

Fahrenheit (°F)	Celsius (°C)
200°F	93°C
300°F	149°C
350°F	177°C
400°F	204°C
450°F	232°C

Volume

Unit	Equivalent
1 teaspoon (tsp)	1/3 tablespoon (tbsp)
1 tablespoon (tbsp)	3 teaspoons (tsp)
1 cup	16 tablespoons (tbsp)
1 pint (pt)	2 cups
1 quart (qt)	4 cups

Chapter 3

BREAKFAST

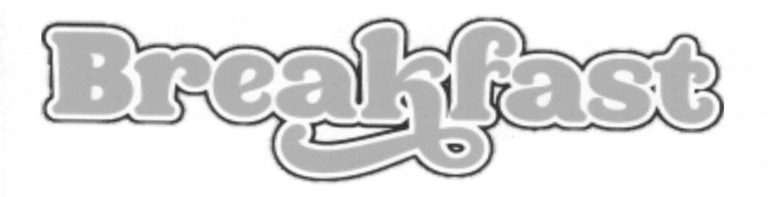

Warm Spiced Oatmeal

This simple yet satisfying oatmeal is infused with warming spices to awaken your digestive fire (agni) and provide gentle nourishment for your body and mind. It's a perfect way to start your day, especially during colder months or for those with a Vata imbalance.

Prep: 5 Mins | Cook: 10 Mins | Total: 15 Mins | Serves: 1

Ingredients

- 1/2 cup rolled oats
- 1 cup milk (dairy or plant-based)
- 1/4 teaspoon ground cinnamon
- 1/4 teaspoon ground cardamom
- 1/8 teaspoon ground ginger
- Pinch of ground nutmeg
- Pinch of salt
- 1 tablespoon chopped nuts (almonds, walnuts, or pecans)
- 1 tablespoon seeds (pumpkin, sunflower, or chia)
- 1 teaspoon ghee (optional)
- 1-2 teaspoons sweetener of choice (honey, maple syrup, or jaggery)

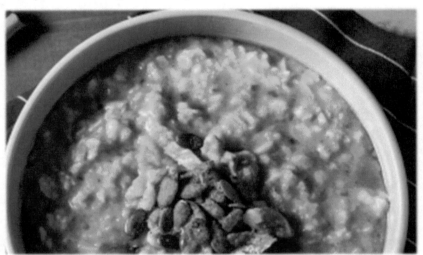

Preparation

1. Combine oats, milk, spices, and salt in a small saucepan.
2. Bring to a boil, then reduce heat and simmer for 5-7 minutes, or until oats are cooked through, stirring occasionally.
3. If using ghee, melt it in a separate pan and pour over the cooked oatmeal.
4. Stir in sweetener of choice and top with chopped nuts and seeds.

Nutrition

Calories: 300 | Protein: 10g | Fat: 8g | Carbs: 35g | Fiber: 7g

Ayurvedic Considerations

- Vata: This warming and nourishing breakfast is ideal for balancing Vata dosha.
- Pitta: Reduce or omit the ginger to avoid excess heat. You can also add a pinch of cooling fennel seeds.
- Kapha: Use less milk or water and reduce the amount of sweetener.

Chickpea Flour Pancakes

These savory pancakes, also known as besan chilla, are a protein-rich, gluten-free breakfast option that is both grounding and easy to digest.

Prep: 15 mins | Cook: 20 mins | Total: 35 mins | Serves: 3

Ingredients

- 1 cup chickpea flour (besan)
- 1/2 teaspoon cumin seeds
- 1/2 teaspoon coriander seeds
- 1/2 teaspoon turmeric powder
- 1/4 teaspoon black pepper
- 1/4 teaspoon rock salt or Himalayan pink salt
- 1/4 cup chopped cilantro
- 1/4 cup chopped mint
- 1/4 cup chopped onion (optional)
- 1/4 cup chopped vegetables like grated carrots, zucchini, or spinach (optional)
- Ghee or coconut oil for cooking

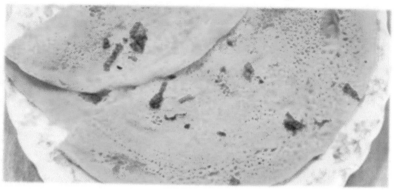

Preparation

1. In a dry skillet, lightly toast the cumin and coriander seeds until fragrant. Remove from heat and grind into a powder.
2. In a mixing bowl, combine the chickpea flour, toasted spice powder, turmeric, black pepper, salt, cilantro, mint, and any optional vegetables.
3. Gradually add water (about 1.5 cups) and whisk until you have a smooth batter, similar to crepe batter consistency. Let the batter rest for 10-15 minutes.
4. Heat a non-stick skillet over medium heat and add a teaspoon of ghee or coconut oil.
5. Pour a ladleful of batter onto the skillet and spread it into a thin circle.
6. Cook for 2-3 minutes on each side, or until golden brown and cooked through.
7. Repeat with the remaining batter, adding more ghee or oil as needed.

Nutrition

Calories: 200 | Protein: 11g | Fat: 7g | Carbs: 25g | Fiber:8g

Ayurvedic Considerations

- This recipe is suitable for all doshas, but it is particularly balancing for Vata due to its warming and grounding properties.
- Chickpea flour is a good source of protein and fiber, making it a satisfying and nourishing breakfast option.
- The spices used in this recipe are digestive aids and help to balance Agni (digestive fire).
- The addition of fresh herbs adds flavor and prana (life force) to the dish

Coconut Milk Chia Seed Pudding

A nourishing and easy-to-digest breakfast option, perfect for balancing Vata and Pitta doshas. The combination of coconut milk, chia seeds, and cardamom provides a cooling and calming effect, while the fresh fruit adds sweetness and vibrancy.

Total: 5 minutes + 8 hours (overnight soaking) | Serves: 2

Ingredients

- 1 cup full-fat coconut milk
- 1/4 cup chia seeds
- 1/2 teaspoon ground cardamom
- 1 tablespoon maple syrup or honey (optional)
- Fresh berries or chopped fruit for topping (mango, banana, pomegranate, etc.)
- Chopped nuts or seeds for added crunch (optional)

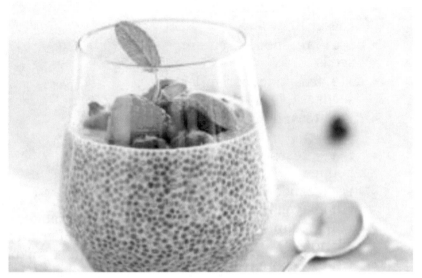

Preparation

1. In a jar or bowl, whisk together the coconut milk, chia seeds, and cardamom.
2. If desired, add maple syrup or honey for sweetness.
3. Cover and refrigerate for at least 8 hours or overnight, allowing the chia seeds to absorb the liquid and create a pudding-like consistency.
4. Before serving, stir well and top with fresh fruit, chopped nuts, or seeds.

Nutrition

Calories: 250 | Protein: 5g | Fat: 20g | Carbs: 15g | Fiber: 10g

Ayurvedic Considerations

- Coconut milk: Cooling and nourishing, balances Vata and Pitta doshas.
- Chia seeds: Cooling and hydrating, rich in fiber and omega-3 fatty acids.
- Cardamom: Digestive aid, promotes oral health, balances Vata and Kapha doshas.
- Fresh fruit: Provides natural sweetness and antioxidants.
- Nuts and seeds: Add healthy fats and protein.
- Note: For a Vata-balancing option, you can warm the coconut milk slightly before adding the chia seeds

Spiced Carrot and Ginger Muffins

The combination of grated carrots, warming ginger, and aromatic spices creates a symphony of flavors that awaken the senses and nourish the body.

Prep: 15 mins | Cook: 30 mins | Total: 45 mins | Serves: 12 muffins

Ingredients

- 2 cups almond flour
- 1 teaspoon baking powder
- 1/2 teaspoon baking soda
- 1/2 teaspoon salt
- 1 teaspoon ground cinnamon
- 1/2 teaspoon ground ginger
- 1/4 teaspoon ground cardamom
- 1/4 teaspoon ground nutmeg
- 1/4 teaspoon ground cloves
- 1/2 cup grated jaggery or coconut sugar
- 1/2 cup melted ghee or coconut oil (for a dairy-free alternative)
- 2 large eggs
- 1 cup grated carrots
- 1/2 cup chopped walnuts or pecans (optional)

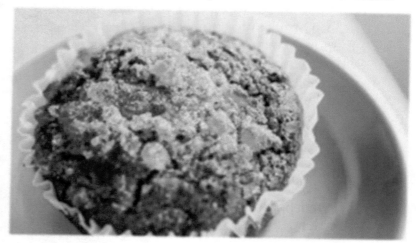

Preparation

1. Preheat the oven to 350°F (175°C). Line each cup of your muffin tin with a paper liner to get it ready for baking.
2. In a large bowl, whisk together the almond flour, baking powder, baking soda, salt, and spices.
3. In a separate bowl, whisk together the jaggery, ghee, and eggs until well combined.
4. Combine the wet ingredients with the dry mixture, stirring gently until just blended.
5. Gently fold in the grated carrots and nuts, if desired.
6. Spoon the batter into the muffin cups, making sure to distribute it evenly.
7. Bake for 25-30 minutes, or until a toothpick inserted into the center emerges clean.
8. Allow the muffins to cool in the pan for a few minutes, then transfer them to a wire rack to finish cooling completely.

Nutrition

Calories: 180 | Fat: 14g | Carbs: 10g | Protein: 5g | Fiber: 3g

Ayurvedic Considerations

1. The combination of warming spices like ginger, cinnamon, and cardamom helps to balance Vata and Kapha doshas.
2. The sweetness of jaggery or coconut sugar provides a nourishing and grounding effect.
3. Carrots are a good source of beta-carotene, which is beneficial for eye health and immunity.

Golden Milk Smoothie

A nourishing and anti-inflammatory Ayurvedic breakfast that harmonizes the doshas and provides sustained energy.

Prep: 5 mins | Total: 5 mins | Serves: 1

Ingredients

- 1 cup milk of choice (almond, coconut, or oat milk are ideal)
- 1/2 teaspoon turmeric powder
- A quarter (1/4) teaspoon ginger powder (or a 1-inch piece of fresh ginger, peeled and grated)
- 1/4 teaspoon cinnamon powder
- Pinch of black pepper
- 2-3 pitted dates (soaked in warm water for 10 minutes for easier blending)
- Optional: a pinch of cardamom or nutmeg for extra flavor

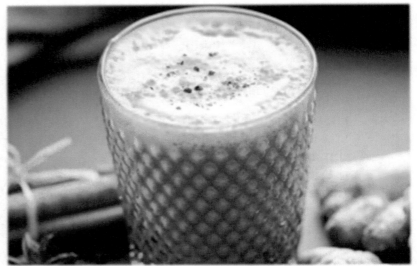

Preparation

1. Combine all ingredients in a blender.
2. Blend until smooth and creamy.
3. Pour into a glass and enjoy warm or cold.

Nutrition

Calories: 250 | Protein: 5g | Fat: 8g | Carbs: 30g | Fiber: 3g

Ayurvedic Considerations

- This smoothie is balancing for all three doshas, but particularly beneficial for Vata and Kapha due to its warming and grounding properties.
- Turmeric is a potent anti-inflammatory and antioxidant.
- Ginger aids digestion and circulation.
- Cinnamon helps regulate blood sugar levels.
- Black pepper enhances the absorption of turmeric.
- Dates provide natural sweetness and energy.

Sweet Potato and Coconut Flour Pancakes

The natural sweetness of the sweet potato harmonizes beautifully with the gentle warmth of the spices, enhanced by the light and fluffy texture imparted by coconut flour.

Prep: 10 mins | Cook: 15 mins | Total: 25 mins | Serves: 2

Ingredients

- One (1) cup mashed sweet potato (cooked and cooled)
- 1/4 cup coconut flour
- 2 eggs
- 1/4 cup unsweetened almond milk or coconut milk
- 1/4 teaspoon ground cinnamon
- 1/4 teaspoon ground ginger
- 1/8 teaspoon ground nutmeg
- Pinch of salt
- Ghee or coconut oil for cooking

Ayurvedic Consideration

- Vata: The warming spices (cinnamon, ginger, nutmeg) help to balance Vata's cold and dry qualities. The sweet potato provides grounding and nourishment.
- Pitta: The coconut milk and sweet potato offer cooling properties to balance Pitta's heat.
- Kapha: The use of coconut flour and spices helps to lighten the dish and promote digestion, which is beneficial for Kaph

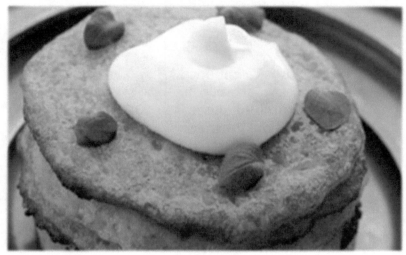

Preparation

1. In a mixing bowl, combine the mashed sweet potato, coconut flour, eggs, almond milk, cinnamon, ginger, nutmeg, and salt. Mix until well combined.
2. Heat a skillet over medium heat and add a small amount of ghee or coconut oil.
3. Spoon 1/4 cup of batter onto the skillet to make each pancake. Cook for about 2 to 3 minutes on each side, or until both sides are golden brown and the pancakes are thoroughly cooked.
4. Serve warm with a drizzle of honey or maple syrup, and additional toppings like berries, sliced banana, or a dollop of coconut yogurt.

Nutrition

Calories: 185 | Carbs: 15g | Protein: 9g | Fat: 6g | Fiber: 2.5g

Ayurvedic Quinoa Bowl

This vibrant bowl combines fluffy quinoa with colorful sautéed vegetables, creamy avocado, and a perfectly poached egg. The addition of Ayurvedic spices like turmeric and cumin enhances digestion and adds depth of flavor.

Prep: 10 mins | Cook: 20 mins | Total: 30 mins | Serves: 1

Ingredients

- 1/2 cup quinoa, rinsed
- 1 cup water or vegetable broth
- 1 tablespoon ghee or coconut oil
- 1/2 cup chopped vegetables (broccoli, carrots, zucchini, etc.)
- 1/4 teaspoon turmeric powder
- 1/4 teaspoon cumin powder
- Pinch of salt
- 1/2 avocado, sliced
- 1 egg
- 1 tablespoon white vinegar
- Fresh cilantro or parsley for garnish (optional)

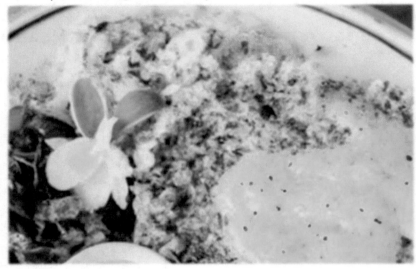

Preparation

1. Combine quinoa and water or broth in a saucepan. Bring to a boil, then reduce heat and simmer, covered, for 15 minutes or until the liquid is absorbed.
2. While the quinoa simmers, gently heat either ghee or coconut oil in a skillet over medium heat. Add the vegetables and spices. Sauté until tender-crisp, about 5 minutes.
3. Poach the egg: Fill a small saucepan with 2 inches of water and add vinegar. Bring to a simmer. Crack the egg into a small bowl and gently slip it into the simmering water. Simmer for 3-4 minutes until the whites are fully set, leaving the yolk perfectly soft and runny.
4. Fluff the cooked quinoa with a fork. Top with the sautéed vegetables, sliced avocado, and poached egg. Garnish with fresh herbs if desired.

Nutrition

Calories: 450 | Protein: 18g | Fat: 25g | Carbohydrates: 40g | Fiber: 10g

Spiced Apple and Pear Porridge

A nourishing and warming porridge that gently awakens the digestive system, perfect for balancing Vata dosha in the colder months. The natural sweetness of apples and pears is enhanced by warming spices like cinnamon and cardamom, creating a comforting and satisfying breakfast.

Prep: 10 mins | Cook: 20 mins | Total: 30 mins | Serves: 2

Ingredients

- 1 apple, peeled, cored, and diced
- 1 pear, peeled, cored, and diced
- 1 cup rolled oats
- Two (2) cups water or milk (dairy or plant-based)
- 1/2 teaspoon ground cinnamon
- 1/4 teaspoon ground cardamom
- Pinch of ground nutmeg
- One (1) tablespoon ghee (clarified butter) or coconut oil
- Optional toppings: chopped nuts, seeds, a drizzle of honey or maple syrup

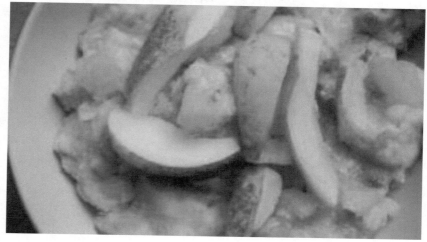

Preparation

1. In a saucepan, combine the diced apples, pears, and water or milk. Bring to a simmer and cook until the fruit is tender, about 10 minutes.
2. Add the oats, cinnamon, cardamom, and nutmeg to the saucepan. Stir well to combine.
3. Continue to cook, stirring occasionally, until the oats are tender and the porridge has thickened, about 10 minutes.
4. Remove from heat and stir in the ghee or coconut oil.
5. Divide the porridge between two bowls and top with your desired toppings.

Nutrition

Calories: 250 | Protein: 7g | Fat: 8g | Carbs: 38g | Fiber: 6g

Ayurvedic Considerations

- This recipe is ideal for Vata dosha due to its warming and grounding properties.
- Pitta individuals can enjoy this dish in moderation, especially during colder months.
- Kapha individuals can reduce the amount of sweetener and add a pinch of ginger for a more balancing effect.
- This porridge is tridoshic when prepared with milk and can be adapted to be suitable for all doshas with slight modifications.

Banana and Almond Butter Smoothie

This creamy and nourishing smoothie is a perfect Ayurvedic breakfast, providing sustained energy and balancing Vata dosha due to its warm and grounding properties. The sweetness of the banana, protein from the almond butter, and warming spices create a harmonious blend that promotes digestion and satiation.

Prep: 5 mins | Total: 5 mins | Serves: 1

Ingredients

- 1 ripe banana (preferably at room temperature)
- 1 tablespoon almond butter (unsweetened)
- 1 cup warm milk (dairy or plant-based)
- 1/4 teaspoon ground cinnamon
- Pinch of nutmeg (optional)

Ayurvedic Considerations

- This smoothie is ideal for Vata dosha due to its warm, grounding, and nourishing qualities.
- For Pitta dosha, you can reduce or omit the banana and add a handful of leafy greens like spinach or kale for a cooling effect.
- For Kapha dosha, use less banana and almond butter, and add a pinch of ginger or black pepper for a warming and stimulating effect

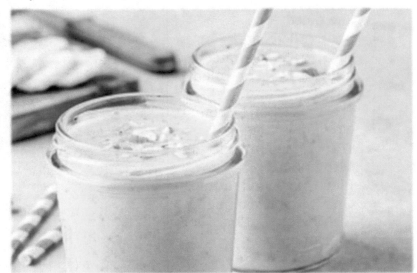

Preparation

1. Combine all ingredients in a blender.
2. Blend until smooth and creamy.
3. Pour into a glass and enjoy immediately.

Nutrition

Calories: 290 | Protein: 13g | Fat: 11g | Carbs: 19g | Fiber: 3g

Spiced Carrot and Zucchini Bread

This moist and flavorful bread is a delightful Ayurvedic breakfast option. Packed with nourishing vegetables and warming spices, it provides sustained energy and supports digestion.

Prep: 15 mins | Cook: 50 mins | Total: 1 hr. - 1 hr. 5 mins | Serves: 8

Ingredients

- Two (2) cups grated zucchini (about 2 medium zucchini)
- One (1) cup of grated carrot (approx. 2 medium carrots)
- 1 cup almond flour
- 1/2 cup arrowroot powder or tapioca starch
- 1/4 cup melted coconut oil or ghee
- 1/3 cup maple syrup or honey
- 2 eggs
- 1 teaspoon baking powder
- 1 teaspoon baking soda
- 1 teaspoon ground cinnamon
- 1/2 teaspoon ground ginger
- 1/4 teaspoon ground nutmeg
- Pinch of sea salt

Ayurvedic Considerations

- Vata: This bread is grounding and warming, making it a good choice for Vata individuals.
- Pitta: The spices used in this recipe are cooling and balancing for Pitta.
- Kapha: Enjoy in moderation, as the

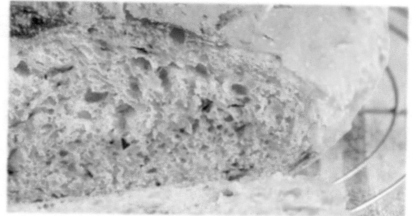

sweetness and density can increase Kapha.

Preparation

1. Preheat oven to 350°F (175°C). Grease a loaf pan.
2. In a spacious mixing bowl, blend together freshly grated zucchini and carrot.
3. In another bowl, thoroughly mix almond flour, arrowroot powder, baking powder, baking soda, cinnamon, ginger, nutmeg, and salt using a whisk.
4. In another bowl, whisk together melted coconut oil, maple syrup, and eggs.
5. Combine the liquid ingredients with the dry ingredients until they are just incorporated together.
6. Fold in the grated zucchini and carrot.
7. Pour the batter evenly into the loaf pan that has been prepared with a lining, then bake it in the oven for 45 to 50 minutes, or until a toothpick inserted into the center of the loaf emerges without any batter sticking to it.
8. Allow the bread to rest in the pan for about 10 minutes to cool slightly before slicing and serving it.

Nutrition

Calories: 150 | Fat: 9g | Carbs: 14g | Protein: 4g | Fiber: 3g | Sugar: 8g

Oatmeal with Eggs and Greens

Start your day with a comforting breakfast bowl brimming with protein, fiber, and vital nutrients to fuel your morning.

Prep: 5 mins | Cook: 15 mins | Total: 20 mins | Serves: 1

Ingredients

- 1/2 cup rolled oats
- 1 cup vegetable broth (or bone broth for non-vegetarians)
- Pinch of salt
- 1 tablespoon ghee or coconut oil
- 1/2 cup chopped kale or spinach
- 1 egg
- Optional toppings: chopped fresh herbs, black pepper, a drizzle of ghee

Ayurvedic Considerations

- This dish is tridoshic, meaning it is suitable for all three doshas (Vata, Pitta, and Kapha).
- Eggs are a good source of protein and choline, supporting brain health.
- Spices like black pepper can aid digestion and boost metabolism.

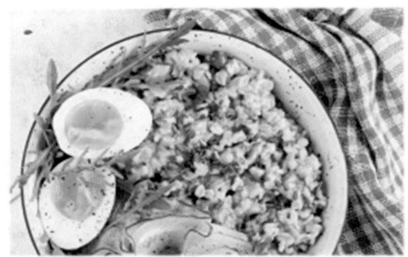

Preparation

1. In a small saucepan, combine oats, broth, and salt. Bring to a boil, then reduce heat to low and simmer for 10-12 minutes, or until oats are cooked through and liquid is absorbed.
2. While the oats are cooking, heat ghee or coconut oil in a small skillet over medium heat. Add the chopped greens and sauté until wilted, about 2-3 minutes.
3. In a separate skillet, fry or poach the egg to your desired doneness.
4. To prepare, transfer the cooked oatmeal into a bowl. Layer it with the wilted greens and egg, then season with black pepper and a pinch of salt to taste. Sprinkle with freshly chopped herbs and optionally add a touch of ghee for added flavor.

Nutrition

Calories: 342 | Protein: 17.5g | Fat: 18g | Carbs: 27g | Fiber: 6g

Buckwheat Pancakes with Berries and Yogurt

A nourishing and grounding breakfast option, these gluten-free pancakes are made with protein-rich buckwheat flour and topped with antioxidant-rich berries and probiotic yogurt. This combination supports healthy digestion, provides sustained energy, and balances all three doshas.

Prep: 10 mins | Cook: 15 mins | Total: 25 mins | Serves: 2

Ingredients

- 1 cup buckwheat flour
- 1 cup milk of choice (almond milk or coconut milk)
- 1 egg
- One (1) tbsp. of ghee (clarified butter) or coconut oil
- 1/2 teaspoon ground cinnamon
- 1/4 teaspoon ground cardamom
- Pinch of salt
- 1 cup mixed berries (blueberries, raspberries, strawberries)
- 1/2 cup plain yogurt
- Optional: Honey or maple syrup (added sweetness)

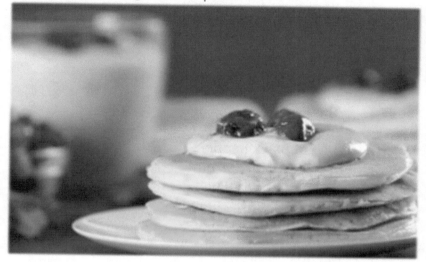

Preparation

1. In a bowl, whisk together buckwheat flour, milk, egg, ghee or coconut oil, cinnamon, cardamom, and salt until smooth.
2. Warm a skillet or griddle over medium heat, lightly greasing it with oil.
3. Pour about a quarter (1/4) cup of pancake batter onto the heated skillet. Cook until bubbles form on the surface, then flip the pancake and continue cooking until both sides are golden brown and cooked through.
4. Top each pancake with berries and a dollop of yogurt. Drizzle a touch of honey or maple syrup for extra sweetness, if preferred.

Nutrition

Calories: 350 | Protein: 12g | Fat: 18g | Carbs: 35g | Fiber: 6g | Sugar: 10g

Ayurvedic Considerations

- Buckwheat is a warming and grounding grain, balancing for Vata dosha.
- Berries are rich in antioxidants and cooling, balancing for Pitta dosha.
- Yogurt is a probiotic food that aids digestion and supports gut health.

Golden Milk Chia Seed Pudding

This creamy and comforting Golden Milk Chia Seed Pudding is packed with anti-inflammatory spices and nourishing ingredients, making it the perfect Ayurvedic breakfast or snack to balance your doshas and promote overall well-being.

Prep: 5 mins | Total: 5 mins + overnight soaking | Serves: 2

Ingredients

- One (1) of cup unsweetened almond milk (or any plant-based milk)
- 1/4 teaspoon turmeric powder
- 1/8 teaspoon ground ginger
- 1/8 teaspoon ground cinnamon
- Pinch of black pepper
- 1/4 teaspoon ground cardamom (optional)
- 1/2 teaspoon maple syrup or honey (optional)
- 1/4 cup chia seeds
- Toppings: chopped nuts (almonds, cashews), seeds (pumpkin, sunflower), berries, shredded coconut

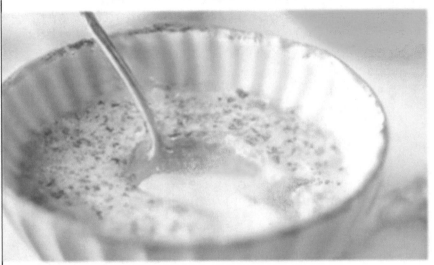

Preparation

1. In a jar or bowl, whisk together the almond milk, turmeric, ginger, cinnamon, black pepper, cardamom (if using), and sweetener (if using).
2. Mix thoroughly until the chia seeds are evenly incorporated.
3. Cover and refrigerate overnight or for at least 4 hours, until the pudding thickens.
4. Before serving, stir the pudding again and add your desired toppings.

Nutrition

Calories: 200 | Protein: 5g | Fat: 12g | Carbohydrates: 18g

Ayurvedic Considerations

- Naturally, this recipe is gluten-free, dairy-free, and also aligns with vegan.
- The warming spices like turmeric, ginger, and cinnamon help to balance Vata and Kapha doshas.
- Chia seeds are a good source of fiber and omega-3 fatty acids, promoting digestive health.
- Almond milk is a cooling and nourishing alternative to dairy milk, suitable for all doshas.
- Feel free to adjust the sweetness and spice level to your personal preferences.

Savory Mung Bean Pancakes

These protein-rich pancakes are a delicious and satisfying Ayurvedic breakfast option. Mung beans are easy to digest and balancing for all three doshas. The warming spices like cumin, coriander, and turmeric aid digestion and boost metabolism.

Prep: 15 mins | Cook: 20 mins | Total: 35 mins | Serves: 4

Ingredients

- 1 cup whole mung beans
- 1/4 cup chopped cilantro
- 1/2 teaspoon cumin seeds
- 1/2 teaspoon coriander seeds
- 1/2 teaspoon turmeric powder
- 1/4 teaspoon black pepper
- Pinch of asafoetida (hing)
- Rock salt to taste
- Ghee or coconut oil for cooking

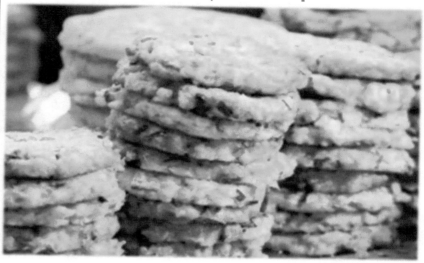

Preparation

1. Rinse the mung beans thoroughly and soak them overnight in plenty of water.
2. Drain the soaked mung beans and grind them into a smooth batter using a blender or food processor.
3. Add chopped cilantro, cumin seeds, coriander seeds, turmeric powder, black pepper, asafoetida, and salt to the batter. Mix well.
4. Heat a non-stick pan or griddle over medium heat, then add a teaspoon of either ghee or coconut oil to the pan.
5. Pour a ladleful of batter onto the pan, and then carefully spread them out to form a thin circle.
6. Cook for 2-3 minutes on each side, or until golden brown and cooked through.
7. Serve hot with chutney or yogurt.

Nutrition

Calories: 200 | Protein: 10g | Fat: 5g | Carbs: 25g | Fiber: 5g

Ayurvedic Considerations

- Mung beans are considered tridoshic, offering balance and support across all three doshas in Ayurveda.
- Cumin, coriander, and turmeric are warming spices that aid digestion.

Sweet Potato Breakfast Bowl

This breakfast bowl is perfect for balancing Vata dosha. The sweet potato provides natural sweetness and fiber, while the quinoa offers protein and complex carbohydrates. The nuts and seeds add healthy fats and crunch, and the drizzle of honey or maple syrup provides a touch of sweetness and warmth.

Prep: 15 mins | Cook: 30 mins | Total: 45 mins | Serves: 2

Ingredients

- 1 large sweet potato, peeled and cubed
- 1/2 cup quinoa, rinsed
- 1 cup water
- 1 tablespoon ghee or coconut oil
- 1/4 teaspoon each: ground cumin, coriander, cinnamon
- Pinch of salt
- 1/4 cup chopped walnuts or almonds
- 1/4 cup pumpkin seeds
- 1 tablespoon honey or maple syrup (optional)

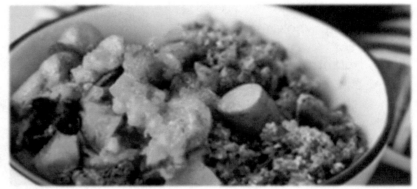

Preparation

1. Preheat oven to 400°F (200°C).
2. Toss sweet potato cubes with ghee or coconut oil, cumin, coriander, cinnamon, and salt.
3. Spread sweet potato cubes on a baking sheet and roast for 25-30 minutes, or until tender and slightly caramelized.
4. While sweet potatoes are roasting, combine quinoa and water in a saucepan. Bring to a boil, then reduce heat to low, cover, and simmer for 15 minutes, or until the water is absorbed and quinoa is cooked.
5. Divide cooked quinoa between two bowls. Top with roasted sweet potato cubes, walnuts or almonds, and pumpkin seeds.
6. Drizzle a touch of sweetness with honey or maple syrup, if you prefer.

Nutrition

Calories: 350 | Protein: 10g | Carbs: 39g | Fat: 15g | Fiber: 10g

Ayurvedic Considerations

- This recipe is naturally gluten-free and can be easily adapted to be vegan by using maple syrup instead of honey.
- The combination of sweet potato and quinoa is grounding and nourishing, making it ideal for Vata dosha.
- The warming spices, such as cumin, coriander, and cinnamon, help to kindle digestion and balance Vata and Kapha.

Spiced Coconut Milk Porridge

This creamy and comforting porridge is a nourishing and warming way to start your day. The coconut milk provides healthy fats and electrolytes, while the oats offer fiber and sustained energy. The warming spices like cinnamon, ginger, and cardamom not only add flavor but also aid digestion and boost metabolism.

Prep: 5 mins | Cook: 10 mins | Total: 15 mins | Serves: 1

Ingredients

- 1/2 cup rolled oats
- 1 cup full-fat coconut milk (canned or homemade)
- 1/4 teaspoon ground cinnamon
- 1/4 teaspoon ground ginger
- Pinch of ground cardamom
- Pinch of sea salt
- 1 tablespoon chopped nuts (almonds, cashews, or walnuts)
- 1 tablespoon mixed seeds (pumpkin, sunflower, or hemp)
- Optional: 1 teaspoon maple syrup or honey (to taste)
- Optional: Fresh berries for garnish

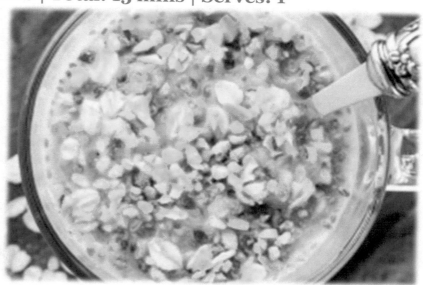

Preparation

1. In a small saucepan, combine oats, coconut milk, cinnamon, ginger, cardamom, and salt.
2. Bring to a boil, then reduce heat to low and simmer for 8-10 minutes, or until oats are cooked through and the porridge has thickened.
3. For added sweetness, mix in maple syrup or honey according to your taste preferences.
4. Pour porridge into a bowl and top with chopped nuts, seeds, and fresh berries (optional).

Nutrition

Calories: 350 | Protein: 8g | Fat: 20g | Carbs: 35g | Fiber: 6g

Ayurvedic Considerations

- This recipe is suitable for all doshas, but particularly beneficial for Vata and Pitta.
- Adjust the spices according to your dosha:
- Vata: Increase warming spices like ginger and cardamom.
- Pitta: Consider reducing ginger and incorporating cooling spices such as fennel or coriander for a balanced flavor profile.
- Kapha: Use all spices in moderation.
- If you are Kapha-dominant, use less coconut milk or substitute with almond milk.

Buckwheat and Berry Smoothie

This breakfast creates a balanced and nourishing breakfast that's perfect for balancing Vata dosha. Buckwheat is a warming and grounding grain, while berries are cooling and packed with antioxidants. Banana adds natural sweetness and creaminess. The smoothie is easy to digest and provides sustained energy throughout the morning.

Prep: 5 mins | Cook: 15 mins | Total: 20 mins | Serves: 1

Ingredients

- 1/2 cup cooked buckwheat groats (See notes for cooking instructions)
- 1 cup mixed berries (fresh or frozen)
- 1 ripe banana
- 1 cup milk of choice (almond, coconut, or oat milk are good options)
- 1/2 teaspoon ground cinnamon
- Pinch of cardamom powder
- Pinch of nutmeg powder

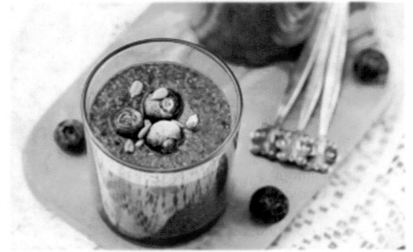

Preparation

1. If using frozen berries, thaw them slightly before blending.
2. Combine all ingredients in a blender.
3. Blend until smooth and creamy.
4. Pour into a glass and enjoy immediately.

Notes

- To cook buckwheat groats: Rinse 1/2 cup groats thoroughly. Begin by combining 1 cup of water with the ingredients in a saucepan. Bring the mixture to a boil, then lower the heat and let it simmer for about 15 minutes, or until it becomes tender. Let cool slightly before using.
- Adjust the sweetness of the smoothie by adding more or less banana, depending on your preference.
- To increase your protein intake, consider stirring in a tablespoon of nut butter or protein powder for an added boost.
- Garnish with additional berries, nuts, or seeds.

Nutrition

Calories: 350 | Protein: 10g | Carbs: 45g | Fat: 10g | Fiber: 12g

LUNCH

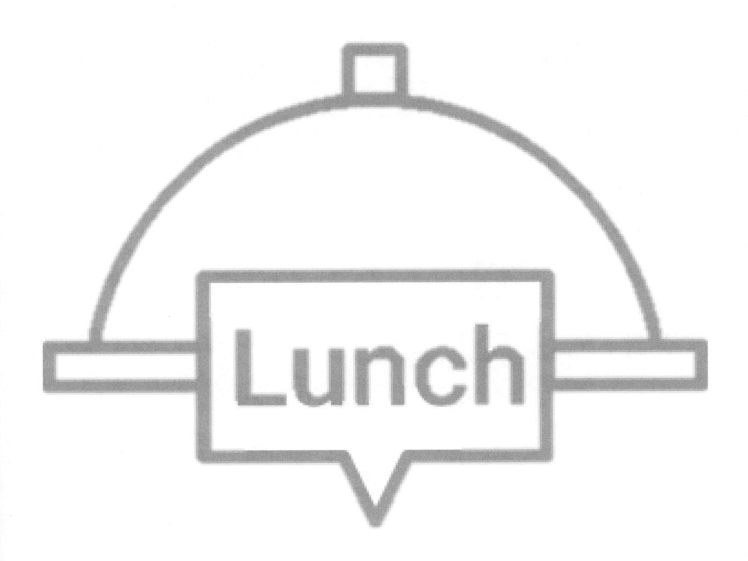

Kitchari

Kitchari is a simple yet nourishing one-pot meal that is considered a staple in Ayurveda. It's made with basmati rice, mung beans, ghee, warming spices, and vegetables. This dish is easy to digest, balances all three doshas, and is particularly beneficial for women's health due to its grounding and nourishing qualities.

Prep: 15 mins | Cook: 45 mins | Total: 1 hr. | Serves: 4

Ingredients

- 1 cup basmati rice, rinsed
- 1/2 cup split yellow mung beans, rinsed
- 1 tablespoon ghee
- 1 teaspoon cumin seeds
- 1 teaspoon coriander seeds
- 1 teaspoon turmeric powder
- 1/2 teaspoon grated fresh ginger
- Pinch of asafoetida (hing)
- 6 cups water
- 1 cup chopped vegetables (carrots, zucchini, cauliflower, etc.)
- Salt to taste
- Fresh cilantro for garnish

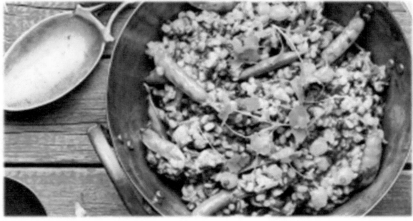

Preparation

- Warm the ghee in a large pot over medium heat until it's melted and ready to use.
- Add cumin and coriander seeds. When they start to sizzle, add turmeric powder, ginger, and asafoetida. Sauté for 30 seconds.
- Add the rice and mung beans, and stir to coat with the spices.
- Add the water to the pot and bring it to a rolling boil.
- Reduce heat to low, cover, and simmer for 30-40 minutes, or until the rice and mung beans are tender.
- Add the chopped vegetables and cook until they are soft, about 10 minutes.
- Season with salt to taste.
- Garnish with fresh cilantro and serve warm.

Nutrition

Calories: 300 | Protein: 12g | Fat: 10g | Carbs: 31g | Fiber: 9g

Ayurvedic Tips

- To address Vata imbalance, incorporate extra ghee and enrich your dishes with warming spices such as ginger and black pepper.
- For Pitta imbalance, use less ghee and add cooling vegetables like zucchini and cilantro.
- For Kapha imbalance, use less ghee and add pungent spices like mustard seeds and black pepper.

Red Lentil Soup with Coconut Milk and Turmeric

This recipe combines the grounding and warming properties of red lentils with the creamy richness of coconut milk and the anti-inflammatory benefits of turmeric. The addition of warming spices like cumin, coriander, and ginger enhances digestion and adds depth of flavor.

Prep: 10 mins | Cook: 30 mins | Total: 40 mins | Serves: 4

Ingredients

- 1 cup red lentils, rinsed
- 1 tablespoon ghee or coconut oil
- 1 onion, chopped
- 2 cloves garlic, minced
- 1-inch piece fresh ginger, grated
- 1 teaspoon ground cumin
- 1 teaspoon ground coriander
- 1/2 teaspoon ground turmeric
- 1/4 teaspoon cayenne pepper (optional)
- 4 cups vegetable broth
- 1 (14-ounce) can full-fat coconut milk
- 1/4 cup chopped fresh cilantro
- Salt and black pepper to taste
- Lime wedges for serving

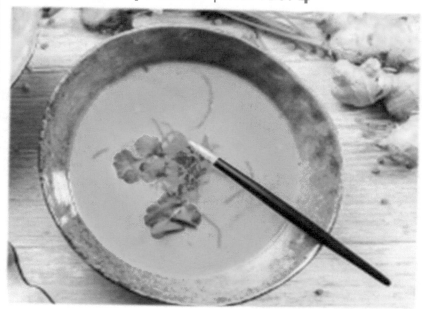

Preparation

1. In a large pot over medium heat, heat up the ghee or coconut oil. Stir in the onion and cook until it becomes soft, approximately 5 minutes.
2. Add the garlic, ginger, cumin, coriander, turmeric, and cayenne pepper (if using) and cook for 1 minute more, stirring constantly.
3. Next, toss the lentils into the pot along with the vegetable broth. Bring to a boil, then reduce heat to low, cover, and simmer for 20-25 minutes, or until the lentils are tender.
4. Stir in the coconut milk and cilantro. Finish by adding salt and black pepper to your liking, adjusting the seasoning as desired.
5. Serve hot with a squeeze of lime juice and additional cilantro, if desired.

Nutrition

Calories: 250 | Protein: 12g | Fat: 15g | Carbs: 20g | Fiber: 8g

Roasted Vegetable salad with Tahini Dressing

This vibrant salad combines the nutty quinoa with the sweetness of roasted vegetables and the creamy richness of tahini dressing. It's a light yet satisfying lunch that aligns with Ayurvedic principles, balancing all three doshas.

Prep: 20 mins | Cook: 30 mins | Total: 50 mins | Serves: 4

Ingredients

- 1 cup quinoa, rinsed
- 2 cups water or vegetable broth
- 1 sweet potato, peeled and cubed
- 1 zucchini, diced
- 1 red bell pepper, diced
- 1 yellow bell pepper, diced
- 1 red onion, thinly sliced
- 2 tablespoons olive oil
- Salt and pepper to taste
- 1/4 cup chopped fresh parsley or cilantro
- Tahini Dressing
- 1/4 cup tahini
- 2 tablespoons lemon juice
- 2 tablespoons water
- 1 clove garlic, minced (optional)
- Optional: One (1) tsp. of honey or maple syrup (to taste)
- Salt and pepper to taste

Preparation

1. Preheat oven to 400°F (200°C).
2. Combine quinoa and water/broth in a saucepan. Bring to a boil, then reduce heat and simmer covered for 15 minutes, or until the liquid is absorbed. Fluff the grains with a fork and allow them to cool before using.
3. Toss the diced vegetables with olive oil, salt, and pepper. Spread evenly on a baking sheet and roast for 20-25 minutes until tender and lightly caramelized.
4. While the vegetables roast, whisk together all the dressing ingredients in a small bowl until smooth and creamy. Adjust consistency with water as needed.
5. In a large bowl, combine the cooked quinoa, roasted vegetables, chopped herbs, and tahini dressing. Toss gently to coat.

Ayurvedic Considerations

- Quinoa: This ancient grain is a complete protein and a good source of fiber, making it a balanced and nourishing choice for all doshas.
- Vegetables: Colorful vegetables provide essential vitamins, minerals, and antioxidants. Choose vegetables that are in season and suitable for your dosha.
- Tahini: Made from sesame seeds, tahini is a good source of healthy fats and protein. It is considered warming and grounding, making it especially beneficial for Vata dosha.
- Spices: Use warming spices like cumin, coriander, or ginger to enhance digestion and balance Vata dosha.

Nutrition

Calories: 350 | Protein: 12g | Fat: 18g | Carbs: 35g | Fiber: 8g

Sweet Potato and Chickpea Curry

This warming and nourishing curry is packed with flavor and nutrients. Sweet potatoes provide grounding energy, while chickpeas offer protein and fiber. The coconut milk adds richness and creaminess, and the fragrant spices aid digestion and provide anti-inflammatory benefits.

Prep: 15 mins | Cook: 30 mins | Total: 45 mins | Serves: 4

Ingredients

- 1 tablespoon ghee or coconut oil
- 1 onion, chopped
- 2 cloves garlic, minced
- 1-inch piece ginger, grated
- 1 teaspoon ground turmeric
- 1 teaspoon ground cumin
- 1/2 teaspoon ground coriander
- 1/4 teaspoon cayenne pepper (optional)
- 2 sweet potatoes, peeled and cubed
- One (1) can (15 ounces) chickpeas, drained and rinsed
- 1 can (14 ounces) full-fat coconut milk
- 1 cup vegetable broth
- 1/2 teaspoon salt, or to taste
- Fresh cilantro leaves for garnish (optional)

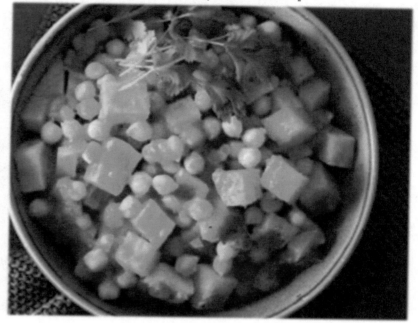

Preparation

1. Heat the ghee or coconut oil in a large pot or Dutch oven over medium heat.
2. Sauté the onion until it softens, which should take around 5 minutes.
3. Add the garlic, ginger, turmeric, cumin, coriander, and cayenne pepper (if using), and cook for 1 minute more.
4. Stir in the sweet potatoes, chickpeas, coconut milk, vegetable broth, and salt.
5. Bring to a boil, then reduce heat to low, cover, and simmer for 25-30 minutes, or until the sweet potatoes are tender.
6. For a thicker curry, you can mash some of the chickpeas against the side of the pot if you like.
7. Taste and adjust seasonings as needed.
8. Garnish with fresh cilantro leaves, if desired, and serve warm.

Nutrition

Calories: 350 | Protein: 10g | Fat: 18g | Carbs: 35g | Fiber: 10g

Spiced Lentil Wraps with Avocado and Greens

A nourishing and satisfying Ayurvedic lunch option, these wraps combine protein-rich lentils with healthy fats from avocado and the freshness of leafy greens. The warming spices aid digestion and provide a delightful flavor profile.

Prep: 15 mins | Cook: 20 mins | Total: 35 mins | Serves: 2

Ingredients

- 1 cup red lentils
- 1 tablespoon ghee or coconut oil
- 1 teaspoon cumin seeds
- 1/2 teaspoon turmeric powder
- 1/4 teaspoon coriander powder
- 1/4 teaspoon chili powder (optional)
- Pinch of asafoetida (hing)
- 1/4 cup chopped cilantro
- 1/4 cup chopped mint
- Salt to taste
- 4 whole wheat or gluten-free tortillas
- 1 ripe avocado, sliced
- 2 cups mixed leafy greens (spinach, kale, arugula)

Ayurvedic Considerations

- o Vata-Pacifying: The warmth of the cooked lentils and spices helps balance Vata dosha.
- o Pitta-Pacifying: The cooling properties of cilantro and mint help balance Pitta dosha.
- o Kapha-Pacifying: The spices and the light nature of the leafy greens help balance Kapha dosha.

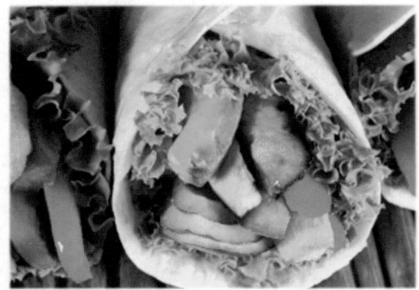

Preparation

1. Rinse the lentils and cook them in 2 cups of water until soft.
2. While the lentils are cooking, heat the ghee or coconut oil in a pan. Add cumin seeds and let them splutter.
3. Add turmeric powder, coriander powder, chili powder (if using), and asafoetida. Sauté for a few seconds.
4. Stir in the cooked lentils and mix thoroughly. Season with salt and add chopped cilantro and mint.
5. Warm the tortillas in a dry skillet or microwave until they're heated through.
6. Fill each tortilla with the spiced lentils, avocado slices, and leafy greens. Roll and enjoy!

Nutrition

Calories: 450 | Protein: 18g | Fat: 20g | Carbs: 47g | Fiber: 15g

Vegetable Curry & Coconut Rice

Prep: 15 mins | Cook: 30 mins | Total: 45 mins | Serves: 4

Ingredients

- Curry
- 1 tablespoon coconut oil or ghee
- 1 onion, chopped
- 2 cloves garlic, minced
- 1-inch piece ginger, grated
- 1 teaspoon turmeric powder
- 1 teaspoon cumin powder
- 1 teaspoon coriander powder
- 1/2 teaspoon garam masala
- 1/4 teaspoon cayenne pepper (optional)
- 1 can (14 ounces) coconut milk
- 1 cup vegetable broth
- 1 head broccoli, cut into florets
- 1 red bell pepper, chopped
- 1 zucchini, chopped
- 1 cup chopped cauliflower
- One (1) can (15 ounces) chickpeas, drained and rinsed
- Salt and pepper to taste
- Fresh cilantro, chopped (for garnish)
- Coconut Rice
- 1 cup basmati rice
- 1 can (14 ounces) coconut milk
- 1 1/2 cups water
- Pinch of salt

Preparation

1. Rinse the rice thoroughly. In a saucepan, mix together the rice, coconut milk, water, and salt. Bring the mixture to a boil, then lower the heat, cover, and let it simmer for 15-20 minutes, or until the rice is tender and the liquid has been absorbed.
2. While the rice is cooking, heat the oil or ghee in a large pot or Dutch oven over medium heat. Toss in the onion and sauté for about 5 minutes, or until it softens. Stir in the garlic, ginger, and spices (turmeric, cumin, coriander, garam masala, cayenne) and cook for 1 minute more.
3. Pour in the coconut milk and vegetable broth, then add the broccoli, bell pepper, zucchini, cauliflower, and chickpeas. Bring to a simmer, then lower the heat and cook for 15-20 minutes until the vegetables are tender. Add a pinch of salt and pepper to season to your taste.
4. Fluff the coconut rice with a fork and serve alongside the vegetable curry. Garnish with fresh cilantro.
5. Nutrition
6. Calories: 350 | Fat: 18g | Carbs: 35g | Protein: 10g | Fiber: 8g

Ayurvedic Considerations

- This dish is tridoshic, meaning it is suitable for all three doshas.
- The warming spices help balance Vata dosha.
- The cooling coconut milk helps balance Pitta dosha.
- The variety of vegetables and fiber help balance Kapha dosha.
- Use seasonal vegetables for optimal freshness and nutritional value.
- Adjust the spices to your liking and dosha type.

Lentil and Spinach Soup with Lemon and Ginger

The combination of ginger and lemon adds a lively, tangy taste that helps with digestion and promotes detoxification. This soup is suitable for all doshas, especially Vata and Pitta.

Prep: 10 mins | Cook: 25 mins | Total: 35 mins | Serves: 4

Ingredients

- 1 cup red lentils, rinsed
- 4 cups vegetable broth
- 1 tablespoon ghee or coconut oil
- 1 teaspoon cumin seeds
- 1 teaspoon grated fresh ginger
- 1/2 teaspoon turmeric powder
- 1/4 teaspoon black pepper
- 4 cups fresh spinach, roughly chopped
- Juice of 1/2 lemon
- Salt to taste
- Fresh cilantro leaves for garnish (optional)

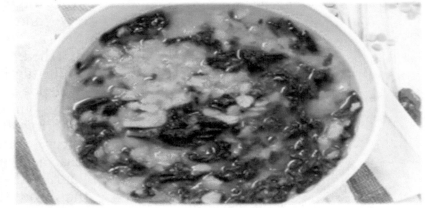

Preparation

1. In a large pot over medium heat, warm up the ghee or coconut oil. Add the cumin seeds and allow to sizzle briefly for a few seconds.
2. Stir in the grated ginger and cook for 1 minute until it becomes fragrant. Then, gently stir in the powdered turmeric and black pepper.
3. Add the red lentils and vegetable broth to the pot. Bring to a boil, then reduce heat to low, cover, and simmer for 15-20 minutes or until the lentils are tender.
4. Stir in the chopped spinach and cook for an additional 2-3 minutes until wilted.
5. Take off the heat and stir in the lemon juice, seasoning with salt to taste.
6. Serve hot, garnished with fresh cilantro leaves if desired.

Nutrition

Calories: 200 | Protein: 12g | Fat: 5g | Carbs: 25g | Fiber: 10g

Note

- o Vata: Increase the amount of ghee or oil, and add a pinch of hing (asafoetida) for its grounding properties.
- o Pitta: Reduce the amount of ginger, and add a cooling herb like cilantro or mint.
- o Kapha: Reduce the amount of oil or ghee, and use less salt.

Quinoa Tabbouleh Salad

It's a perfect Ayurvedic lunch option, as it's easy to digest, cooling, and balancing for all doshas.

Prep: 15 mins | Cook: 20 mins | Total: 35 mins | Serves: 4

Ingredients

1 cup quinoa, rinsed
- 2 cups water
- 1 cucumber, seeded and diced
- 1-pint cherry tomatoes, halved
- 1/2 cup chopped fresh parsley
- 1/4 cup chopped fresh mint
- 1/4 cup extra-virgin olive oil
- Juice of 1 lemon
- 1/4 teaspoon sea salt
- 1/4 teaspoon black pepper

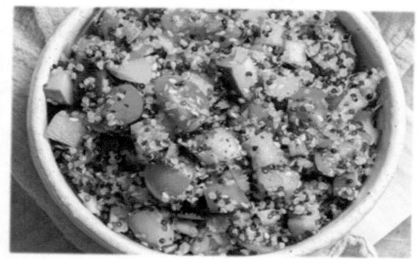

Preparation

1. Combine quinoa and water in a saucepan. Bring the mixture to a boil, then lower the heat, cover, and let it simmer for 15 minutes, or until the quinoa absorbs all the water and becomes fluffy.
2. Combine olive oil, lemon juice, salt, and pepper in a small bowl and whisk together.
3. In a large bowl, mix together parsley, the cucumber, cooked quinoa, mint, and tomatoes. Drizzle the dressing over the salad and mix well until everything is evenly coated.
4. Let the salad cool in the refrigerator for at least 30 minutes before serving. This allows the flavors to meld.

Nutrition

Calories: 250 | Protein: 8g | Fat: 12g | Carbs: 28g | Fiber: 5g

Ayurvedic Considerations

- Dosha Balance: This salad is tridoshic, meaning it's suitable for all dosha types.
- Cooling: The cucumber and herbs have a cooling effect, making this salad ideal for warm weather or for those with excess Pitta.
- Digestive Aid: The lemon juice and herbs help stimulate digestion.
- Nutrient-Dense: Quinoa is a complete protein and provides essential nutrients like iron and magnesium.

Sweet Potato and Black Bean Burger

The sweetness of the sweet potato complements the earthiness of the black beans, while warming spices like cumin and coriander add depth and complexity.

Prep: 20 mins | Cook: 25 mins | Total: 45 mins | Serves: 4

Ingredients

- 2 medium sweet potatoes, baked and mashed
- One (1) can (15 ounces) black beans, rinsed and drained
- 1/2 cup rolled oats
- 1/4 cup chopped cilantro
- 1/4 cup chopped walnuts, finely chopped (optional)
- 1 tablespoon olive oil or ghee
- 1 teaspoon ground cumin
- 1 teaspoon ground coriander
- 1/2 teaspoon turmeric powder
- 1/4 teaspoon cayenne pepper (optional)
- Salt and black pepper to taste
- 4 whole-wheat buns

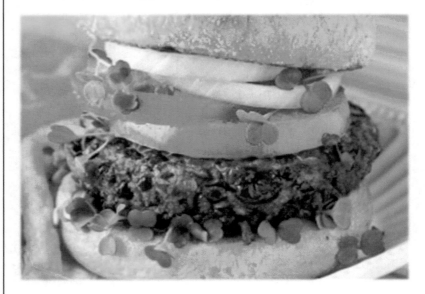

Preparation

1. In a large bowl, combine the mashed sweet potatoes, black beans, oats, cilantro, walnuts (if using), and spices.
2. Continuously stir until all ingredients are evenly mixed.
3. Form the mixture into 4 equal-sized patties.
4. Heat the olive oil or ghee in a skillet over medium heat.
5. Cook the patties for 4-5 minutes per side, or until golden brown and heated through.
6. Serve the yummy burgers on whole-wheat buns with toppings of your choice.

Ayurvedic Considerations

- Sweet Potatoes: Sweet potatoes are grounding and nourishing, making them an excellent choice for balancing Vata dosha.
- Black Beans: Black beans are a protein-rich legume that helps to balance Kapha dosha.
- Oats: Oats are a warming and grounding grain that helps to balance Vata and Pitta doshas.

Nutrition

Calories: 350 | Protein: 15g | Fat: 12g | Carbs: 45g | Fiber: 10g

Lentil Vegetable Fritters with Yogurt Dip

The warming spices and cooling yogurt dip create a balanced and satisfying Ayurvedic lunch.

Prep: 20 mins | Cook: 15 mins | Total: 35 mins | Serves: 4

Ingredients

- 1 cup red lentils, rinsed and drained
- 1/2 cup grated carrots
- 1/2 cup grated zucchini
- 1/4 cup chopped cilantro
- 1/4 cup chopped onion
- 1 tablespoon grated ginger
- 1 teaspoon cumin seeds
- 1 teaspoon coriander powder
- 1/2 teaspoon turmeric powder
- 1/4 teaspoon salt
- Pinch of black pepper
- 1/4 cup chickpea flour (besan)
- Ghee or coconut oil, for frying
- Yogurt Dip
- 1 cup plain yogurt (homemade is best)
- 1/4 cup chopped cucumber
- 1 tablespoon chopped mint
- 1/2 teaspoon cumin powder
- Salt and pepper to taste

Preparation

1. In a saucepan, combine the lentils with 2 cups of water. Bring to a boil, then reduce heat and simmer for 15-20 minutes until lentils are tender but firm. Drain any excess water.
2. In a large bowl, combine the cooked lentils, grated carrots, zucchini, cilantro, onion, ginger, cumin seeds, coriander powder, turmeric powder, salt, and black pepper. Mix well.
3. Gradually add the chickpea flour to the lentil mixture, mixing until you have a thick batter. If the batter is too dry, add a tablespoon of water at a time until you reach the desired consistency.
4. Heat ghee or coconut oil in a skillet over medium heat. Drop spoonfuls of the batter onto the skillet and flatten slightly. Sauté for 3-4 minutes per side until golden brown and done.
5. While the fritters are cooking, combine all the yogurt dip ingredients in a small bowl. Mix well and season to taste.
6. Serve the warm lentil fritters with the cooling yogurt dip.

Nutrition

Calories: 250 | Protein: 12g | Fat: 10g | Carbs: 28g | Fiber: 8g

Ayurvedic Considerations

1. This recipe is tridoshic, meaning it is suitable for all three doshas (Vata, Pitta, and Kapha).
2. Red lentils are easy to digest and provide grounding energy.
3. The combination of vegetables provides a variety of nutrients.
4. Warming spices like cumin, coriander, and turmeric aid digestion and balance Vata and Kapha.
5. The cooling yogurt dip balances Pitta and provides probiotics for gut health.

Roasted Vegetable Salad with Turmeric Tahini Dressing

Prep: 20 mins | Cook: 40 mins | Total: 60 mins | Serves: 4

Ingredients

Vegetables

- One (1) medium head of cauliflower, cut into florets
- One (1) medium head of broccoli, cut into florets
- 2 medium carrots, peeled and chopped
- 1 red onion, cut into wedges
- One (1) bell pepper (any color), cut into chunks
- 1 cup Brussels sprouts, halved
- 1 tablespoon olive oil
- Salt and pepper to taste
- Chickpeas
- One (1) can (15 ounces), drained and rinsed chickpeas,
- 1 teaspoon olive oil
- 1/2 teaspoon turmeric powder
- 1/4 teaspoon cumin powder
- 1/4 teaspoon coriander powder
- Pinch of cayenne pepper (optional)

Turmeric Tahini Dressing

- 1/4 cup tahini
- 2 tablespoons lemon juice
- 1 tablespoon olive oil
- 1 tablespoon water
- 1 teaspoon turmeric powder
- 1/2 teaspoon ground cumin
- 1/4 teaspoon ground ginger
- Salt and pepper to taste

Preparation

1. Preheat oven to 400°F (200°C).
2. Toss vegetables with olive oil, salt, and pepper. Arrange on a baking sheet and roast for 30-40 minutes until tender and slightly browned.
3. While vegetables are roasting, toss chickpeas with olive oil, turmeric, cumin, coriander, and cayenne pepper (if using). Arrange on a separate baking sheet and this time, roast for 20 minutes, or until crispy.
4. In a small bowl, whisk together tahini, lemon juice, olive oil, water, turmeric, cumin, ginger, salt, and pepper until smooth.
5. In a large bowl, combine roasted vegetables, chickpeas, and drizzle with turmeric tahini dressing. Toss to coat.

Nutrition

Calories: 350 | Protein: 12g | Fat: 20g | Carbs: 30g | Fiber: 10g

Ayurvedic Adaptations

- This recipe is naturally aligned with Ayurvedic principles, emphasizing whole, unprocessed ingredients and gentle cooking methods.
- To further balance Vata dosha, you can add a pinch of warming spices like cinnamon or nutmeg to the dressing.
- If Pitta dosha is aggravated, reduce or omit the cayenne pepper.
- For Kapha dosha, use less oil and choose lighter vegetables like broccoli and zucchini.

Quinoa Black Bean Salad with Avocado Dressing

Prep: 15 mins | Cook: 20 mins | Total: 35 mins | Serves: 4

Ingredients

- 1 cup quinoa, rinsed
- 2 cups water
- One (1) can (15 ounces) black beans, rinsed and drained
- 1 cup frozen or fresh corn kernels
- 1 cup cherry tomatoes, halved
- 1/2 cup chopped cilantro
- 1 ripe avocado
- 1/4 cup lime juice
- 1/4 cup extra-virgin olive oil
- 1/4 cup chopped red onion
- 1 clove garlic, minced
- 1/2 teaspoon cumin powder
- 1/4 teaspoon salt
- Pinch of black pepper

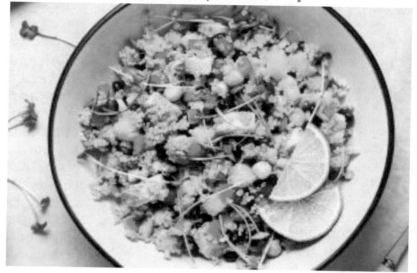

Preparation

1. To start, get a saucepan and mix the quinoa and water, then bring to a boil. Reduce heat to low, cover, and gently simmer for 15-20 minutes until the quinoa is cooked and the water is absorbed. Fluff with a fork, set aside and then, allow it cool.
2. In a blender or food processor, combine the avocado, lime juice, olive oil, red onion, garlic, cumin, salt, and pepper. Blend until smooth and creamy.
3. In a large bowl, combine the cooked quinoa, black beans, corn, cherry tomatoes, and cilantro.
4. Drizzle the prepared avocado dressing on top the salad and toss to coat.
5. Enjoy the salad immediately or chill for later.

Nutrition

Calories: 370 | Protein: 9.5g | Fat: 21g | Carbs: 32.3g | Fiber: 10g

Ayurvedic Considerations

- This quinoa salad is tridoshic, which means it is suitable for all three doshas. However, individuals with a predominantly Kapha constitution may want to reduce the amount of avocado in the dressing.

Chickpea Curry with Spinach and Coconut Milk

Prep: 15 mins | Cook: 25 mins | Total: 40 mins | Serves: 4

Ingredients

- 1 tablespoon coconut oil or ghee
- 1 onion, finely chopped
- 3 cloves garlic, minced
- 1-inch piece ginger, grated
- 1 teaspoon ground turmeric
- 1 teaspoon ground cumin
- 1/2 teaspoon ground coriander
- 1/4 teaspoon cayenne pepper (optional)
- One (1)-14 ounce can diced tomatoes, with their juices
- One (1)-14 ounce can chickpeas, drained and rinsed
- 1 (14 ounce) can full-fat coconut milk
- 4 cups fresh spinach, roughly chopped
- Salt and black pepper to taste
- Fresh cilantro, for garnish (optional)

Preparation

1. Heat the coconut oil or ghee in a large pot or Dutch oven over medium heat. Gently, toss in the onion and sauté for approx. 5 minutes until softened.
2. Add the garlic, coriander, turmeric, ginger, cayenne pepper (if using), and cumin. Stir continuously and cook for approx. 1 minute until fragrant.
3. Stir in the diced tomatoes and their juices. Bring to a simmer and cook, stirring occasionally, for 10 minutes, or until the sauce has thickened slightly.
4. Carefully stir in the chickpeas and coconut milk. Add a touch of salt and pepper to suit your taste.
5. Simmer for 15 minutes, stirring occasionally, until the chickpeas are heated through and the flavors meld.
6. Next, carefully mix in the spinach and cook until wilted, about 2 minutes more.
7. Garnish with fresh cilantro if desired and serve the delicious curry hot.

Nutrition

Calories: 312 | Protein: 11g | Fat: 17g | Carbohydrates: 27g | Fiber: 10g

Ayurvedic Considerations

- This delicious curry is tridoshic, whuch means it is suitable for all three doshas.
- The warming spices, such as turmeric, cumin, and ginger, help to balance Vata and Kapha.
- The coconut milk provides healthy fats that nourish the body and balance Vata.
- The spinach is a good source of iron and other nutrients that support women's health.
- You can adjust the amount of cayenne pepper to suit your taste and dosha type. If you are Pitta dominant, you may want to omit it or use a smaller amount.

Spiced Lentil and Brown Rice Bowl

A nourishing and grounding one-bowl meal, perfect for lunch or a light dinner. Warming spices like cumin, coriander, and turmeric add depth and promote digestion.

Prep: 15 mins | Cook: 30 mins | Total: 45 mins | Serves: 4

Ingredients

- 1 cup brown rice, rinsed
- 1 cup red lentils, rinsed
- 2 cups chopped mixed vegetables (such as carrots, broccoli, cauliflower, zucchini)
- 1 tablespoon ghee or coconut oil
- 1 teaspoon cumin seeds
- 1 teaspoon coriander seeds
- 1/2 teaspoon turmeric powder
- 1/4 teaspoon salt
- Pinch of black pepper
- 2 tablespoons tahini
- Fresh cilantro or parsley for garnish

Ayurvedic Considerations

- This dish is tridoshic, meaning it is suitable for all three doshas (Vata, Pitta, and Kapha).
- Red lentils are a good source of protein and fiber, making them a nourishing and grounding food.
- The combination of cumin, coriander, and turmeric helps to stimulate digestion and reduce inflammation.

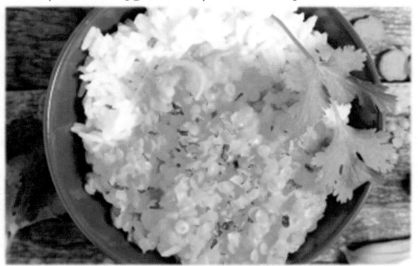

Preparation

1. Combine the rice and lentils in a pot with 3 cups of water. Bring to a boil, then reduce heat to low, cover, and simmer for 25-30 minutes, or until the rice and lentils are tender.
2. While the rice and lentils are cooking, preheat the oven to 400°F (200°C). Toss the chopped vegetables with ghee or coconut oil, salt, and pepper. Arrange on a baking sheet and roast for 20-25 minutes until tender and slightly browned.
3. In a small saucepan, melt the ghee or coconut oil over medium heat. Add the cumin seeds, coriander seeds, turmeric powder, and salt. Sauté for at least 30 seconds until the spices are fragrant.
4. Divide the cooked rice and lentils among four bowls. Top with roasted vegetables and a drizzle of tahini. Garnish with fresh cilantro or parsley.

Nutrition

Calories: 280 | Protein: 13g | Fat: 7g | Carbohydrates: 33g | Fiber: 10g

Roasted Cauliflower and Chickpea Salad

Description: A vibrant and nourishing Ayurvedic salad, balancing Vata and Pitta doshas, featuring roasted cauliflower and chickpeas tossed in a zesty lemon tahini dressing.

Prep: 15 mins | Cook: 30 mins | Total: 45 mins | Serves: 4

Ingredients

- 1 head cauliflower, cut into florets
- One (1) can (15 ounces), drained and rinsed chickpeas
- 1 red onion, thinly sliced
- 2 tablespoons extra-virgin olive oil
- 1 teaspoon ground cumin
- 1/2 teaspoon turmeric powder
- 1/4 teaspoon cayenne pepper (optional, for Pitta)
- Salt and black pepper to taste
- Fresh cilantro, chopped, for garnish
- Lemon Tahini Dressing
- 1/4 cup tahini
- 1/4 cup water
- 3 tablespoons lemon juice
- 2 cloves garlic, minced
- 1/2 teaspoon ground cumin
- Pinch of cayenne pepper (optional, for Pitta)
- Salt to taste

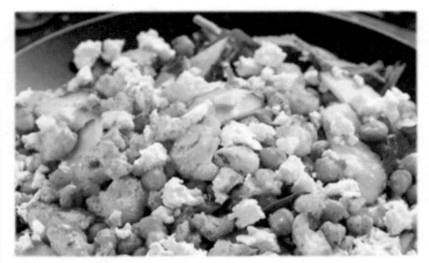

Preparation

1. To start preheat your oven to 400°F (200°C).
2. In a large bowl, toss cauliflower florets, chickpeas, and red onion with olive oil, cumin, turmeric, cayenne (if using), salt, and pepper.
3. Spread the vegetables in a single layer on a baking sheet and roast for 25-30 minutes, or until the cauliflower is tender and slightly browned.
4. While the vegetables are roasting, whisk together all dressing ingredients in a small bowl until smooth and creamy. Adjust seasonings to taste.
5. After the veggies has roasted, allow them cool slightly. Get a large bow and gently toss the roasted veggies with the lemon tahini dressing. Top this with the chopped cilantro and serve warm or at room temperature.

Nutrition

Calories: 295 | Protein: 12g | Fat: 16g | Carbohydrates: 22g | Fiber: 5g

Ayurvedic Considerations

- Suitable for All Doshas: This salad is generally suitable for all doshas, but you can adjust the spices and ingredients to suit your individual needs. For example, reduce or omit the cayenne pepper if you have a Pitta imbalance.

Sweet Potato and Lentil Curry with Coconut Milk

It's a balanced and satisfying Ayurvedic lunch that's easy to digest and provides sustained energy.

Prep: 15 mins | Cook: 40 mins | Total: 55 mins | Serves: 4

Ingredients

- 1 tablespoon ghee or coconut oil
- 1 onion, chopped
- 2 cloves garlic, minced
- 1-inch piece ginger, grated
- 1 teaspoon ground turmeric
- 1 teaspoon ground cumin
- 1/2 teaspoon ground coriander
- 1/4 teaspoon cayenne pepper (optional)
- 1 sweet potato, peeled and cubed
- 1 cup red lentils, rinsed
- 4 cups vegetable broth
- 1 can (13.5 ounces) full-fat coconut milk
- 1/2 cup chopped fresh cilantro
- Salt and pepper to taste

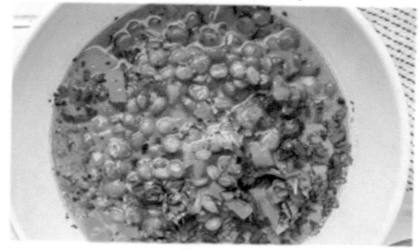

Preparation

1. Warm the ghee or coconut oil in a large pot over medium heat. Then, mix in the onion and sauté until softened, at least 5 minutes.
2. Add the cayenne pepper (if using), ginger, coriander, turmeric, garlic, cumin, and cook for 1 minute more.
3. Add the vegetable broth, sweet potato, and lentils. Bring the mixture to a boil, lower the heat, cover, and cook for 25 minutes, or until the lentils and sweet potatoes becomes tender.
4. Stir in the coconut milk and cilantro. Season with salt and pepper to taste. Simmer for 5 minutes more to allow the flavors to meld.
5. Serve warm over basmati rice or with a side of steamed vegetables.

Nutrition

Calories: 250 | Fat: 11g | Carbs: 23g | Fiber: 12g | Protein: 15g

Ayurvedic Considerations

- This dish is tridoshic, meaning it is suitable for all three doshas.
- Sweet potatoes are grounding and nourishing, balancing Vata dosha.
- Lentils are easy to digest and provide sustained energy, balancing all doshas.

DINNER

dinner

Baked Salmon with Lemon and Dill

A simple, flavorful, and nourishing Ayurvedic dinner that is easy to digest and promotes balance. This dish is rich in omega-3 fatty acids, protein, and vitamin D, all of which are essential for women's health.

Prep: 5 mins | Cook: 20 mins | Total: 25 mins | Serves: 2

Ingredients

- 2 wild-caught salmon fillets (6-8 ounces each)
- 1 organic lemon, sliced
- 1/4 cup fresh dill, chopped
- 1 tablespoon ghee (clarified butter)
- 1/2 teaspoon turmeric powder
- 1/4 teaspoon black pepper
- Pinch of Himalayan salt

Ayurvedic Considerations

- Salmon is a tridoshic food, meaning it is suitable for all three doshas. Because of its warming and grounding properties, it is particularly beneficial to Vata.
- Ghee is a Sattvic food, meaning it promotes clarity, calmness, and balance.
- Turmeric is a powerful anti-inflammatory spice that is balancing for all three doshas.
- Lemon and dill are both cooling and refreshing herbs that are balancing for Pitta

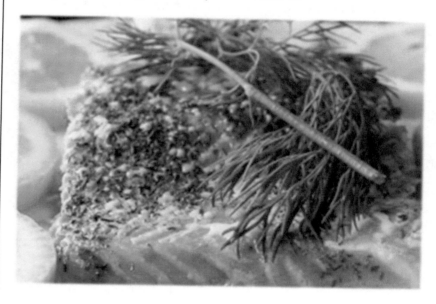

Preparation

1. To begin, first preheat your oven to 400°F (200°C).
2. Rinse salmon fillets with clean water and pat dry using a towel.
3. In a small bowl, combine ghee, turmeric, black pepper, and salt.
4. Rub the ghee mixture over the salmon fillets.
5. Carefully arrange the salmon fillets on a baking sheet lined with parchment paper.
6. Top each fillet with lemon slices and dill.
7. Bake for 15-20 minutes at least, or you noticed the salmon is cooked through and flakes easily with a fork.

Nutrition

Calories: 400 | Protein: 35g | Fat: 25g | Carbs: 10g

Chicken Curry with Coconut Milk and Spinach

This fragrant and flavorful chicken curry is a nourishing and satisfying meal that is perfect for balancing all three doshas. The combination of warming spices, creamy coconut milk, and tender chicken creates a dish that is both comforting and invigorating. The spinach adds a boost of iron and other essential nutrients, making this a complete and wholesome meal.

Prep: 15 mins | Cook: 30 mins | Total: 45 mins | Serves: 4

Ingredients

- One (1) lb. chicken breasts or thighs cut into bite-sized pieces (boneless and skinless)
- 1 tablespoon ghee or coconut oil
- 1 onion, chopped
- 2 cloves garlic, minced
- 1-inch piece ginger, grated
- 1 teaspoon ground turmeric
- 1 teaspoon ground cumin
- 1/2 teaspoon ground coriander
- 1/4 teaspoon cayenne pepper (optional)
- 1 (14-ounce) can full-fat coconut milk
- 1 cup chopped tomatoes
- 4 cups fresh spinach leaves
- Salt and pepper to taste
- Fresh cilantro leaves for garnish

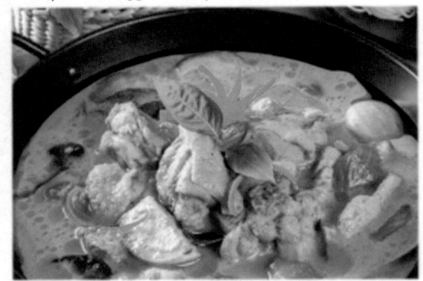

Preparation

1. Warm the ghee or coconut oil in a large skillet over medium heat. Then, mix in the chicken and sauté until browned on all sides. Next is to Remove the chicken from the skillet and set aside.
2. In the same skillet, sauté the garlic, onion, and ginger until the onion softens.
3. Add the cumin, cayenne pepper (if using), turmeric, and., coriander. Stir well to combine.
4. Add the coconut milk and tomatoes and simmer for 10 minutes until the sauce thickens slightly
5. Return the chicken to the skillet and add the spinach. Continue to cook until the chicken is done and the spinach is wilted.
6. Season with salt and pepper to taste. Before serving, top with fresh cilantro leaves for a delightful garnish

Nutrition

Calories: 370 | Protein: 25g | Fat: 20g | Carbs: 10g | Fiber: 5g

Vegetable Stir-Fry with Ginger and Garlic

A vibrant and flavorful stir-fry bursting with colorful vegetables, infused with the warming and digestive properties of ginger and garlic. This dish is light, nourishing, and easy to digest, making it an ideal Ayurvedic dinner.

Prep: 15 mins | Cook: 15 mins | Total: 30 mins | Serves: 2

Ingredient

- 1 tablespoon ghee or coconut oil
- 1 tablespoon grated fresh ginger
- 2 cloves garlic, minced
- 1 medium onion, thinly sliced
- 1 medium carrot, thinly sliced
- 1 bell pepper (any color), thinly sliced
- 1 cup broccoli florets
- 1/2 cup chopped green beans
- 1/4 cup chopped cilantro
- 1/4 teaspoon turmeric powder
- 1/4 teaspoon cumin powder
- 1/4 teaspoon coriander powder
- Salt and black pepper to taste
- Optional: A squeeze of lime juice

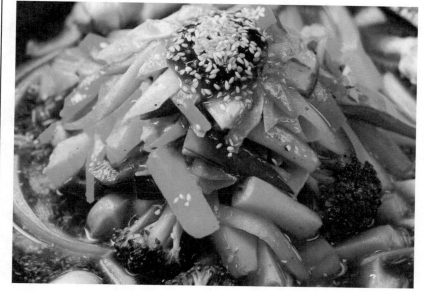

Preparation

1. Heat the ghee or coconut oil in a large skillet or wok over medium heat.
2. Add the ginger and garlic and sauté for 1 minute, or until fragrant.
3. Gently stir in sauté the onion for 2-3 minutes until softened.
4. Add the remaining vegetables and cook for 5-7 minutes, or until tender-crisp, stirring occasionally.
5. Stir in the turmeric, cumin, and coriander powder. Sauté the mixture for another minute until fragrant.
6. Season with salt and pepper to taste.
7. Top with cilantro and a squeeze of lime juice, if desired.
8. Serve hot over cooked quinoa, brown rice, or with roti.

Nutrition

Calories: 230 | Protein: 5g | Fat: 12g | Carbs: 20g | Fiber: 5g

Cauliflower Rice with Turmeric and Peas

Crafted as a wholesome alternative to traditional rice, cauliflower is transformed into a light, nutritious meal. Fragrant spices meld with fresh vegetables in a skillet, creating a dish that's both easy to digest and bursting with flavor.

Prep: 10 mins | Cook: 15 mins | Total: 25 mins | Serves: 2

Ingredients

- 1 head cauliflower, grated or processed into rice-like texture
- 1 tablespoon ghee or coconut oil
- 1/2 teaspoon cumin seeds
- 1/2 teaspoon turmeric powder
- 1/4 teaspoon ground coriander
- 1/4 teaspoon ground ginger
- Pinch of black pepper
- 1/2 cup frozen or fresh peas
- 1/4 cup chopped cilantro
- Salt to taste
- Optional: Chopped nuts for garnish

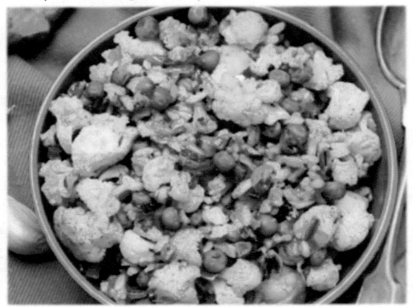

Instructions

1. Begin by heating ghee or coconut oil in a spacious skillet over medium heat.
2. Add cumin seeds and allow them to crackle briefly.
3. Introduce turmeric powder, coriander, ginger, and black pepper, stirring until fragrant, approximately 30 seconds.
4. Incorporate cauliflower rice and peas, cooking for 5-7 minutes until the cauliflower reaches a tender, non-mushy consistency.
5. Season with salt to your liking.
6. Garnish with cilantro and nuts if desired.

Nutrition

Calories: 150 | Carbs: 15g | Protein: 5g | Fat: 8g | Fiber: 5g

Ayurvedic Insights

- Balanced for Doshas: This recipe harmonizes all three doshas (Vata, Pitta, and Kapha), offering easily digestible ingredients and a well-rounded flavor profile.

Sweet Potato and Black Bean Tacos

Where the natural sweetness of roasted sweet potatoes meets protein-rich black beans, enhanced with warming spices for a satisfying meal. A creamy avocado crema adds a cooling touch, balancing flavors while providing essential healthy fats.

Prep: 15 mins | Cook: 25 mins | Total: 40 mins | Serve: 4.

Ingredients

- 2 large sweet potatoes, peeled and cubed
- 1 tbsp olive oil
- 1 tsp cumin
- 1 tsp chili powder
- 1/2 tsp smoked paprika
- 1/4 tsp salt
- 1/4 tsp black pepper
- One (1) (15-oz) can black beans, rinsed and drained
- 8 corn tortillas, warmed
- Avocado Crema
- 1 ripe avocado
- 1/4 cup plain yogurt (or coconut yogurt)
- 1/4 cup chopped cilantro
- 1 tbsp lime juice
- Pinch of salt

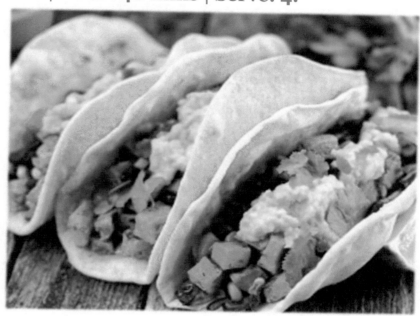

Preparations

1. Preheat oven to 400°F (200°C).
2. Toss sweet potatoes with olive oil, cumin, chili powder, smoked paprika, salt, and pepper. Carefully arrange on a baking sheet and roast for 20-25 minutes until tender.
3. While sweet potatoes roast, prepare avocado crema: Blend avocado, yogurt, cilantro, lime juice, and salt until smooth.
4. Warm tortillas.
5. Fill tortillas with roasted sweet potatoes, black beans, and avocado crema.

Nutrition

Calories: 365 | Protein: 12g | Fat: 17g | Carbs: 39g | Fiber: 10g

Ayurvedic Insights

- Sweet potatoes harmonize all doshas.
- Grounding for Vata, black beans offer balance.
- Cumin and coriander aid digestion.
- Avocado cools and nourishes, ideal for Pitta.

Baked Chicken with Turmeric and Lemon

A dish that marries the anti-inflammatory power of turmeric with the digestive benefits of lemon. This light yet satisfying dinner is both easy to digest and nourishing for the body.

Prep: 15 mins | Cook: 35 mins | Total: 50 mins | Serves: 4

Ingredients

- 4 boneless, skinless chicken breasts (organic, free-range)
- 1 tablespoon turmeric powder
- 1 tablespoon ground cumin
- 1 tablespoon ground coriander
- 1 teaspoon ground black pepper
- 1/2 teaspoon sea salt
- Juice of 1 lemon
- 2 tablespoons ghee or coconut oil, melted

Ayurvedic Insights

- Suitable for all three doshas (Vata, Pitta, and Kapha), this dish is tridoshic.
- Turmeric is renowned for its anti-inflammatory properties, particularly beneficial for Vata and Kapha doshas.
- Lemon aids digestion by stimulating agni (digestive fire) and is balancing for all doshas.
- Ghee or coconut oil are nourishing fats that are easy to digest and beneficial for the body.

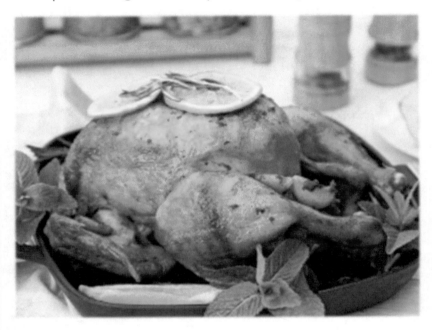

Instructions

1. Begin by preheating your oven to 375°F (190°C).
2. In a small bowl, blend together turmeric, cumin, coriander, black pepper, and salt.
3. Coat the chicken breasts thoroughly with the spice mixture.
4. Arrange the seasoned chicken breasts in a baking dish, then drizzle them with melted ghee or coconut oil and lemon juice.
5. Bake for 30-35 minutes, or until the chicken is fully cooked and the juices run clear.

Nutrition

Calories: 250 | Protein: 30g | Fat: 12g | Carbs: 2g

Ayurvedic Vegetable Biryani

This Ayurvedic-inspired recipe aims to balance the doshas while promoting optimal digestion.

Prep: 30 mins | Cook: 45 mins | Total time: 1 hr. 15 mins | Serves: 4

Ingredients

- one (1) cup basmati rice, soaked for 30 minutes
- 1 tablespoon ghee (clarified butter)
- 1 large onion, thinly sliced
- 2 cloves garlic, minced
- 1-inch piece ginger, grated
- 1 teaspoon cumin seeds
- 1 teaspoon coriander powder
- 1/2 teaspoon turmeric powder
- A quarter (1/4) teaspoon red chili powder (adjust to taste)
- Pinch of saffron strands
- 1 cup mixed vegetables (carrots, cauliflower, peas, beans, potatoes), chopped
- 1/2 cup plain yogurt (whole milk, unsweetened)
- 1 cup chopped fresh cilantro and mint leaves
- Salt to taste
- Lemon wedges, for serving (optional)

Instructions

1. Begin by heating ghee in a large pot or Dutch oven over medium heat. Next, stir in the cumin seeds and let them splutter.
2. Add the onions and cook until they turn golden brown. Incorporate the garlic and ginger, sautéing for another minute.

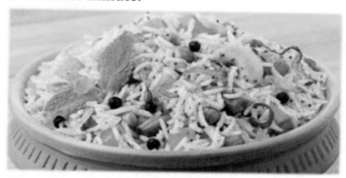

3. Introduce the coriander powder, turmeric powder, and chili powder, sautéing for 30 seconds.
4. Toss in the chopped vegetables and cook until they are slightly tender.
5. Gently, stir in the soaked and drained rice, salt, and saffron-infused milk to the pot.
6. Pour in the yogurt and gently mix all the ingredients together.
7. Cover the pot and simmer on low heat for 20-25 minutes, or until the rice is cooked and the liquid is absorbed.
8. Garnish with chopped cilantro and mint leaves. Serve it hot and enjoy with lemon wedges if desired.

Nutrition

Calories: 315 | Protein: 10g | Fat: 12g | Carbs: 42g | Fiber: 5g

Ayurvedic Insights

- This biryani is designed to be tridoshic, making it suitable for all three doshas (Vata, Pitta, and Kapha) due to its balanced use of spices and vegetables.
- Basmati rice is light on the stomach and supplies sustained energy.
- Yogurt adds a cooling touch and supports digestion.

Salmon with Roasted Vegetables and Tahini Sauce

Indulge in this vibrant and nourishing meal that pairs the rich flavors of salmon with the sweet, earthy notes of roasted vegetables. A creamy tahini sauce infused with Ayurvedic spices completes the dish, making it a balanced and satisfying option for optimal health.

Prep: 15 mins | Cook: 25 mins | Total: 40 mins | Serves: 2

Ingredients

- 1 lb wild-caught, skin-on salmon fillet
- 1 sweet potato, peeled and cubed
- 1 head of broccoli, cut into florets
- 1 red onion, cut into wedges
- 2 tbsp olive oil
- 1 tsp turmeric powder
- 1/2 tsp cumin powder
- 1/4 tsp coriander powder
- Salt and black pepper to taste

Tahini Sauce

- 1/4 cup tahini
- 2 tbsp lemon juice
- 2 tbsp water
- 1 tsp grated ginger
- Pinch of cayenne pepper (optional)
- Salt to taste

Ayurvedic Insights

- This tridoshic dish suits all three doshas (Vata, Pitta, and Kapha).
- Salmon offers omega-3 fatty acids essential for hormonal balance and health.
- Tahini adds healthy fats and protein, enhancing the dish's nutritional profile

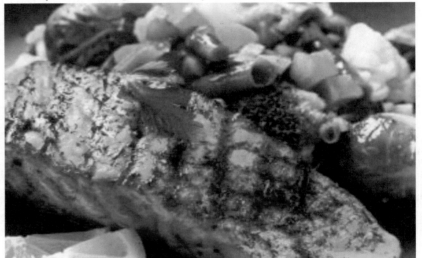

Preparation

1. Preheat your oven to 400°F (200°C).
2. Toss sweet potato, broccoli, and red onion in a large bowl with olive oil. Add turmeric, cumin, coriander, salt, and pepper, mixing well to coat.
3. Spread the vegetables on a baking sheet and roast for 20-25 minutes until tender and slightly browned.
4. While the veggies roast, prepare the tahini sauce by whisking together tahini, lemon juice, water, ginger, cayenne pepper (if using), and salt until smooth.
5. Season the salmon with salt and pepper. Place it on a separate baking sheet and bake for 12-15 minutes, or until fully cooked.
6. Serve by dividing the roasted vegetables among plates, topping with salmon, and drizzling with tahini sauce.

Nutrition

Calories: 500 | Protein: 30g | Fat: 28g | Carbs: 23g | Fiber: 7g

Roasted Vegetable Curry with Tofu or Tempeh

This dish is designed to nourish and balance all three doshas, making it a satisfying meal for any time.

Prep: 20 mins | Cook: 30 mins | Total: 50 mins | Serves: 4

Ingredients

Vegetables

- 1 head cauliflower, cut into florets
- 2 sweet potatoes, peeled and cubed
- 1 red onion, cut into wedges
- 1 bell pepper (any color), chopped
- 1 cup cherry tomatoes
- Protein
- 1 block extra-firm tofu, pressed and cubed (or 1 package tempeh, cubed)

Curry Sauce

- 1 tablespoon coconut oil
- 1 inch ginger, minced
- 3 cloves garlic, minced
- 1 teaspoon ground turmeric
- 1 teaspoon ground cumin
- 1/2 teaspoon ground coriander
- 1/4 teaspoon cayenne pepper (optional)
- 1 (14-ounce) can full-fat coconut milk
- 1/2 cup vegetable broth
- Salt and pepper to taste
- Garnish
- Fresh cilantro, chopped
- Lime wedges

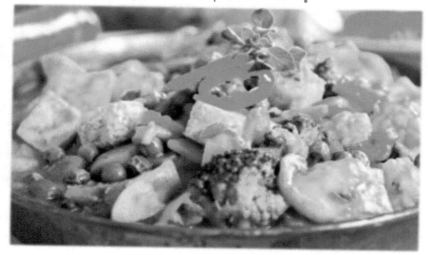

Preparation

1. To begin, first preheat your oven to 400°F (200°C).
2. Toss cauliflower, sweet potatoes, red onion, bell pepper, cherry tomatoes, and cubed tofu or tempeh with a drizzle of coconut oil, salt, and pepper on a baking sheet. Then, roast them for 20-25 minutes until tender and slightly browned.
3. While the vegetables roast, heat coconut oil in a large pot over medium heat. Sauté minced ginger and garlic for 1 minute until fragrant.
4. Stir in turmeric, cumin, coriander, and optional cayenne pepper, cooking for another minute.
5. Pour in coconut milk and vegetable broth, bringing the mixture to a simmer. Season with salt and pepper.
6. Incorporate roasted veggies and tofu/tempeh: Fold in the roasted vegetables and tofu/tempeh into the curry sauce. Simmer for 5 minutes to meld flavors.
7. Spoon curry over brown rice or quinoa. Garnish with fresh cilantro and a squeeze of lime.

Nutrition

Calories: 350 | Protein: 15g | Fat: 20g | Carbs: 25g | Fiber: 10g

One-Pan Lemon Herb Chicken and Vegetables

This easy and satisfying Ayurvedic dinner features tender chicken with vibrant vegetables, all brightened with lemon and herbs. It's a wholesome, balanced meal perfect for any weeknight.

Prep: 15 mins | Cook: 30 mins | Total: 45 mins | Serves: 4

Ingredients

Chicken

- Four (4) boneless, skinless chicken breasts, cut into 1-inch pieces
- 1 tablespoon ghee or coconut oil

Vegetables

- 1 large onion, chopped
- 2 cloves garlic, minced
- 1 head broccoli, cut into florets
- 2 carrots, sliced
- 1 zucchini, sliced

Seasoning

- Half (1/2) cup chopped fresh herbs (such as parsley, dill, and basil)
- 1/4 cup lemon juice
- 1/4 cup vegetable broth (or water)
- Salt and black pepper to taste

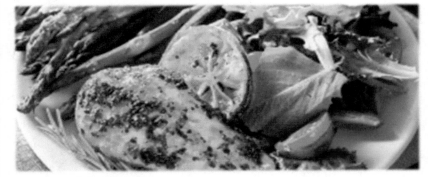

Preparation

1. Preheat oven: Set oven to 400°F (200°C).
2. Cook chicken: In a large oven-safe skillet, melt the ghee or coconut oil over medium heat. Add the chicken pieces and cook for 5-7 minutes, until lightly browned on all sides. Remove and set aside.
3. Sauté vegetables: In the same pan, cook the onion for 5 minutes until softened. Add garlic, broccoli, carrots, and zucchini. After that gently simmer for extra 5-7 mins until vegetables are tender-crisp.
4. Combine and season: Return the chicken to the pan. Mix in the fresh herbs, lemon juice, and vegetable broth. Season with salt and pepper.
5. Bake: Transfer the skillet to the oven and bake for 15-20 minutes, until the chicken is cooked through and vegetables are tender.
6. Serve: Enjoy warm with a side of brown rice or quinoa.

Nutrition

Calories: 350 | Protein: 30g | Fat: 18g | Carbs: 12g | Fiber: 4g | Sugars: 4g

Ayurvedic Adaptations

- Ghee or coconut oil are preferred in Ayurveda for their nourishing and digestive benefits.
- Incorporating warming spices like turmeric and cumin aids digestion and reduces inflammation.
- Herbs such as parsley, dill, and basil enhance flavor and support digestion.

Butternut Squash and Chickpea Curry with Spinach

The sweetness of the squash pairs perfectly with the earthy chickpeas and spinach, while warming spices like ginger and turmeric boost digestion and well-being, making it ideal for balancing Vata dosha in cooler months.

Prep: 15 mins | Cook: 30 mins | Total: 45 mins | Serves: 4

Ingredients

- 1 butternut squash, peeled, seeded, and cubed
- 1 tablespoon coconut oil
- 1 onion, chopped
- 2 cloves garlic, minced
- 1-inch piece of ginger, grated
- 1 teaspoon ground turmeric
- 1 teaspoon ground cumin
- 1/2 teaspoon ground coriander
- 1/4 teaspoon cayenne pepper (optional)
- 1 (14-ounce) can chickpeas, drained and rinsed
- 1 (14-ounce) can full-fat coconut milk
- 1 cup vegetable broth
- 5 ounces baby spinach
- Salt and pepper to taste
- Fresh cilantro leaves for garnish

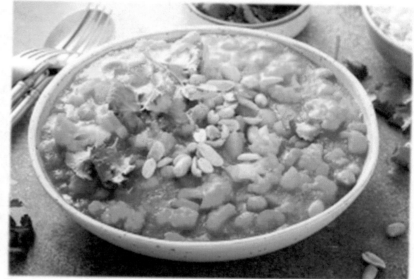

Preparation

1. Heat the oil: Melt the coconut oil in a large pot over medium heat.
2. Cook the onion: Add the chopped onion and sauté until soft, about 5 minutes.
3. Add spices: Stir in garlic, ginger, turmeric, cumin, coriander, and optional cayenne, cooking for another minute while stirring.
4. Combine main ingredients: Add the cubed butternut squash, chickpeas, coconut milk, and vegetable broth. Bring the mixture to a boil, then reduce heat to a simmer for 20 minutes, or until the squash is tender.
5. Add spinach: Stir in the baby spinach and cook until wilted, about 1 minute. Season with salt and pepper to taste.
6. Serve and garnish: Serve hot, garnished with fresh cilantro, over basmati rice or your preferred grain.

Nutrition

Calories: 350 | Fat: 18g | Carbs: 35g | Protein: 12g | Fiber: 10g

Baked Cod with Turmeric and Ginger

This dish features tender cod fillets infused with turmeric and ginger for a flavorful, anti-inflammatory meal. Coconut oil and lime juice enhance the Ayurvedic properties, balancing the doshas and adding a fresh taste.

Prep: 10 mins | Cook: 20 mins | Total: 30 mins | Serves: 2

Ingredients

- 2 cod fillets (about 6 ounces each)
- 1 tablespoon coconut oil, melted
- 1 teaspoon ground turmeric
- 1 teaspoon grated fresh ginger
- 1/2 teaspoon ground cumin
- 1/4 teaspoon black pepper
- 1/2 lime, juiced
- Salt to taste
- Fresh cilantro, chopped (for garnish)

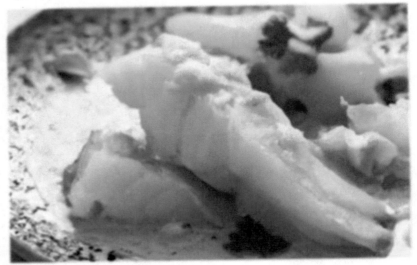

Preparation

1. Preheat the oven: Set to 400°F (200°C).
2. Mix spices: In a small bowl, combine melted coconut oil, turmeric, ginger, cumin, black pepper, lime juice, and salt.
3. Coat the cod: Place cod fillets in a baking dish, then pour and evenly spread the spice mixture over them.
4. Bake: Cook for 15-20 minutes, or until the fish is fully cooked and flakes easily with a fork.
5. Garnish and serve: Top with fresh cilantro and serve immediately.

Nutrition

Calories: 250 | Protein: 30g | Fat: 15g | Carbs: 3g

Ayurvedic Considerations

- Cod: A light, easy-to-digest fish suitable for all doshas, especially Vata and Pitta.
- Turmeric and Ginger: Warming spices that aid digestion and reduce inflammation.
- Coconut Oil: A nourishing fat that helps balance the doshas.
- Lime Juice: Adds a refreshing taste and helps balance Pitta dosha.

Sweet Potato Black Bean Enchiladas

Prep: 30 mins | Cook: 25 mins | Total: 55 mins | Serves: 4

Ingredients

Filling

- 2 large sweet potatoes, peeled and diced
- One (1) can (15 ounces) black beans, rinsed and drained
- 1/2 cup chopped red onion
- 1/2 cup chopped bell pepper (any color)
- 1/4 cup chopped cilantro
- 1 tablespoon chili powder
- 1 teaspoon cumin
- 1/2 teaspoon garlic powder
- 1/4 teaspoon salt
- 1/4 teaspoon black pepper

Sauce

- 1 tablespoon olive oil
- 1/2 cup chopped onion
- 2 cloves garlic, minced
- 1 tablespoon chili powder
- 1 teaspoon cumin
- 1/2 teaspoon smoked paprika
- 1/4 teaspoon cayenne pepper (optional)
- 1 (14.5 ounces) can diced tomatoes, undrained
- 1/2 cup vegetable broth
- 1/4 teaspoon salt
- 1/4 teaspoon black pepper

Other

- 8-12 corn tortillas
- 1/2 cup shredded vegan cheese (optional)

Preparation

1. Prepare Filling: Preheat your oven to 400°F (200°C). Toss the diced sweet potatoes with olive oil, salt, and pepper, then roast for 20-25 minutes until tender.

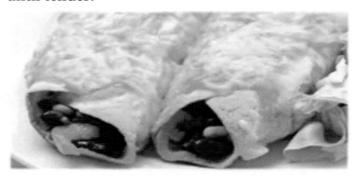

2. Make Sauce: While the potatoes roast, heat olive oil in a saucepan over medium heat. Add the minced garlic and chopped onion and sauté until softened. Add smoked paprika, cumin, chili powder, and cayenne pepper if desired and cook for 1 minute. Finally, mix in the vegetable broth, salt, diced tomatoes, and pepper. After that, bring to a simmer, lower the heat, and cook for 15 another mins.
3. Combine Filling: In a bowl, mix the roasted sweet potatoes, black beans, red onion, bell pepper, cilantro, chili powder, cumin, garlic powder, salt, and pepper.
4. Assemble Enchiladas: Warm the tortillas in a dry skillet or microwave. Dip each tortilla in the prepared sauce, fill with the sweet potato mixture, and roll up. Place in a baking dish.
5. Bake: Drizzle the remaining prepared sauce over the enchiladas and top with vegan cheese if desired, then bake for 17-20 mins until heated through and the cheese is melted.

Nutrition

Calories: 400 | Protein: 12g | Fat: 15g | Carbs: 55g | Fiber: 15g

Creamy Coconut Lentil Curry

This is a nourishing dish that's easy on digestion and perfectly balances all three doshas, offering a particular soothing effect for Vata types.

Prep: 15 mins | Cook: 30 mins | Total: 45 mins | Serves: 4

Ingredients

- 1 cup red lentils, rinsed
- 1 tablespoon coconut oil or ghee
- 1 onion, chopped
- 2 cloves garlic, minced
- 1-inch piece ginger, grated
- 1 teaspoon ground turmeric
- 1 teaspoon ground cumin
- 1/2 teaspoon ground coriander
- 1/4 teaspoon cayenne pepper (optional)
- 1 (14-ounce) can full-fat coconut milk
- 4 cups vegetable broth
- 1 cup chopped vegetables (carrots, sweet potatoes, zucchini, etc.)
- Salt and pepper to taste
- Fresh cilantro for garnish

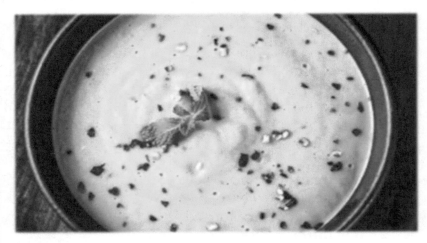

Preparation

1. Sauté Aromatics: Heat coconut oil or ghee in a large pot over medium heat. Stir in already chopped onions and sauté until softened, about 5 mins.
2. Stir in your spices (grated ginger, minced garlic, coriander, turmeric, cumin, and optional cayenne pepper). Cook for another minute, stirring constantly.
3. Combine Ingredients: Add the rinsed lentils, coconut milk, vegetable broth, and chopped vegetables to the pot. Bring the mixture to a boil, then reduce heat to low. Cover and simmer for 25-30 minutes until the lentils are tender and the curry thickens.
4. To Season, add salt and pepper to to suit your taste. Serve hot, garnished with fresh cilantro.

Nutrition

Calories: 350 | Protein: 15g | Fat: 20g | Carbs: 30g | Fiber: 10g

Ayurvedic Considerations

- This recipe is tridoshic, therefore it perfect for all doshas.
- Red lentils are a digestible source of protein and fiber.
- Turmeric and ginger offer warming, anti-inflammatory benefits.
- A variety of vegetables enriches the dish with nutrients and diverse flavors.

SNACKS
Spiced Nuts and Seeds

Enjoy a warm, crunchy snack that's perfect for keeping Vata dosha balanced. This mix of nuts and seeds offers a hearty dose of protein, healthy fats, and essential minerals. The blend of spices not only enhances flavor but also aids digestion and boosts metabolism.

Prep: 5 mins | Cook: 20 mins | Total: 25 mins | Serves: 4

Ingredients

- 1 cup raw almonds
- 1 cup raw cashews
- 1/2 cup pumpkin seeds
- 1/2 cup sunflower seeds
- One (1) tbsp. of ghee (clarified butter) or coconut oil
- 1/2 teaspoon turmeric powder
- 1/2 teaspoon cumin powder
- 1/2 teaspoon coriander powder
- Pinch of cayenne pepper (optional)
- Pinch of salt

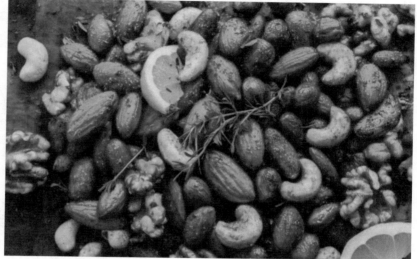

Preparation

1. To begin, preheat your oven to 325°F (165°C).
2. Mix Nuts and Seeds: Combine all the nuts and seeds in a large bowl.
3. Add your oil (ghee or coconut oil) in a small pan, melt them over low heat.
4. Add Spices: Stir turmeric, cumin, coriander, cayenne pepper (if using), and salt into the melted ghee/oil until well blended.
5. Coat Evenly: Pour the spiced ghee/oil over the nuts and seeds, tossing them to ensure even coating.
6. Bake: Spread the mixture in a single layer on a baking sheet lined with parchment paper. Bake for 15-20 minutes, stirring occasionally, until the nuts and seeds are golden brown and fragrant.
7. Cool and Store: Remove from the oven and let cool completely before storing in an airtight container.

Nutrition

Calories: 250 | Protein: 8g | Fat: 15g | Carbs: 5g | Fiber: 5g

Fruit Salad with Mint and Lime

Enjoy a refreshing and vibrant fruit salad that balances all three doshas with its blend of sweet, sour, and astringent flavors. This light and hydrating snack is easy to digest, perfect for any time of day.

Prep: 10 mins | Total: 10 mins | Serves: 4

Ingredients

- 2 cups chopped mango
- 1 cup chopped pineapple
- 1 cup chopped strawberries
- Half (1/2) cup pomegranate arils
- A quarter (1/4) cup chopped fresh mint
- Juice of 1 lime
- Optional: Pinch of cardamom powder

Ayurvedic Considerations

- Vata: The sweetness of the fruit and the warmth of cardamom balance Vata's dry and cold nature.
- Pitta: Cooling mint and lime juice help soothe Pitta's heat.
- Kapha: Astringent pomegranate and digestive lime and mint counterbalance Kapha's heaviness and sluggishness.

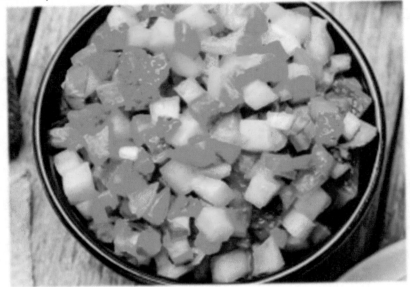

Preparation

1. Combine Fruits: Mix the chopped mango, pineapple, strawberries, and pomegranate arils in a large bowl.
2. Add Mint and Lime: Stir in the chopped mint and lime juice.
3. Toss Gently: Mix gently to combine all ingredients.
4. Sprinkle Cardamom: If desired, add a pinch of cardamom powder for extra warmth and aroma.
5. Serve: Enjoy immediately or chill for an extra refreshing treat.

Nutrition

Calories: 100 | Carbs: 25g | Protein: 1g | Fiber: 4g

Ayurvedic Date and Nut Energy Balls

These nutrient-dense energy balls are a perfect Ayurvedic snack to satisfy your sweet tooth while providing sustained energy. Dates and nuts are known for their nourishing and grounding properties, making them ideal for balancing Vata dosha.

Prep: 15 mins | Total: 15 mins | Serves: 10 balls

Ingredients

- One (1) cup pitted Medjool date (soaked in warm water for 10 minutes)
- 1/2 cup raw almonds
- 1/2 cup raw walnuts
- 1/4 cup shredded coconut (unsweetened)
- 1 tablespoon ghee
- 1/4 teaspoon cardamom powder
- Pinch of sea salt

Ayurvedic Considerations

- Dosha: Balancing for Vata dosha.
- Taste: Primarily sweet, with a hint of astringent from the nuts and a touch of pungent from the cardamom.
- Benefits: Provides sustained energy, nourishes the nervous system, promotes healthy digestion, and satisfies sweet cravings.

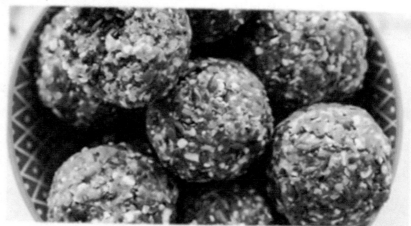

Preparation

1. Drain the soaked dates and discard the water.
2. In a food processor, combine the almonds and walnuts and pulse until finely chopped.
3. In a food processor, combine the shredded coconut, cardamom powder, dates, ghee, and salt.
4. Process until the mixture forms a sticky dough that holds together.
5. Roll the dough into little balls approximately an inch in diameter.
6. If desired, roll the balls in additional shredded coconut.
7. You can refrigerate these balls in an airtight jar for up to two weeks.

Nutrition

Calories: 100 | Protein: 2g | Fat: 6g | Carbs: 12g | Fiber: 2g

Avocado and Egg Toast

Enjoy a wholesome and balanced Ayurvedic snack that combines healthy fats, protein, and fiber. This version of avocado toast features warming spices and a perfectly cooked egg for a satisfying meal.

Prep: 5 mins | Cook: 7 mins | Total: 12 mins | Serves: 1

Ingredients

- 1 slice whole-grain or sourdough bread
- 1/2 ripe avocado
- 1 large egg
- 1/4 teaspoon ghee or coconut oil
- Pinch of sea salt
- Pinch of black pepper
- Pinch of turmeric
- Pinch of cumin
- Optional: Chopped cilantro or fresh herbs for garnish

Ayurvedic Considerations

- o Dosha Suitability: Beneficial for all doshas, particularly grounding and nourishing for Vata.
- o Healthy Fats: Ghee or coconut oil supports digestion and hormonal balance.
- o Warming Spices: Turmeric and cumin enhance warmth and aid digestion.
- o Customization: Adjust spices according to personal taste and dosha type.

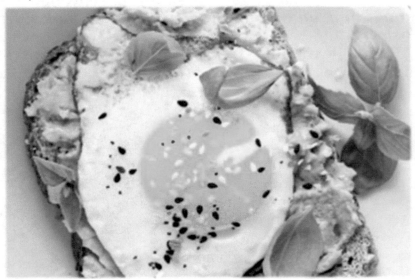

Preparation

1. To begin, first toast your bread to the desired crispness.
2. Heat your oil (ghee or coconut oil) in a small skillet over medium heat. Crack the egg into the skillet and cook it to your preference (sunny-side up, over easy, or scrambled).
3. While the egg cooks, mash the avocado in a bowl. Mix in the salt, pepper, turmeric, and cumin.
4. Spread the prepared seasoned avocado on the toasted bread. Top with the cooked egg.
5. Optionally, sprinkle with chopped cilantro or fresh herbs.

Nutrition

Calories: 350 | Fat: 22g | Carbs: 20g | Protein: 13g | Fiber: 8g

Ayurvedic Spiced Popcorn

This light and airy snack satisfies cravings while balancing all three doshas. The warming spices aid digestion and the ghee provides a nourishing base.

Prep: 5 mins | Cook: 5 mins | Total: 10 mins | Serves: 2-4

Ingredients

- 1/4 cup popcorn kernels
- 1 tablespoon ghee (clarified butter)
- 1/2 teaspoon turmeric powder
- 1/2 teaspoon cumin powder
- 1/4 teaspoon coriander powder
- Pinch of black pepper
- Pinch of Himalayan salt

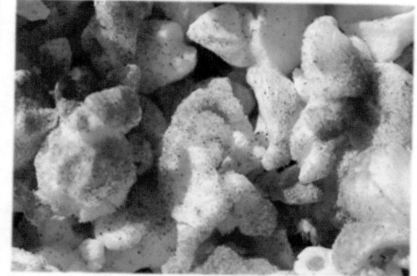

Preparation

1. Heat your ghee in a large-sized pot over medium heat.
2. Add the quarter popcorn kernels and gently cover the pot.
3. Shake the pot gently until the popping slows down.
4. Take the pot off from the heat and place popcorn in a large bowl.
5. Get a medium-sized bowl and then combine the spices and salt.
6. Sprinkle the mixed spices over the popcorn generously and shake vigorously to coat evenly.
7. Serve warm.

Nutrition

Calories: 150 | Fat: 10g | Carbs: 15g | Protein: 3g

Ayurvedic Considerations

- Vata: The warmth of the spices and the grounding quality of ghee help to balance Vata.
- Pitta: The cooling properties of coriander and the anti-inflammatory benefits of turmeric help to balance Pitta.
- Kapha: The lightness of the popcorn and the digestive properties of cumin and pepper help to balance Kapha.

Apple Slices with Almond Butter

This quick and delicious snack is ideal for balancing Vata dosha, combining sweet, astringent, and grounding flavors. Apples provide fiber and antioxidants, while almond butter offers healthy fats and protein.

Prep: 5 mins | Total: 5 mins | Serves: 1

Ingredients

- 1 organic apple (preferably a sweet variety like Fuji or Honeycrisp)
- 2 tablespoons organic almond butter (unsweetened and unsalted)
- Optional: a sprinkle of cinnamon for added warmth

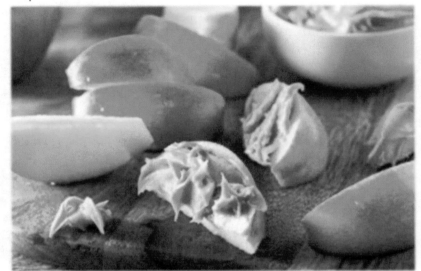

Preparation

1. Wash and Slice: Thoroughly wash the apple. Core it and cut into wedges.
2. Spread Almond Butter: Generously spread almond butter on each apple wedge.
3. Add Cinnamon: Optionally, sprinkle a bit of cinnamon on top for extra warmth.

Nutrition

Calories: 190 | Protein: 5g | Fat: 12g | Carbs: 21g | Fiber: 4g

Ayurvedic Considerations

- Dosha Benefits: Apples are tridoshic, balancing all three doshas, with sweet varieties being especially good for Vata due to their grounding qualities.
- Almond Butter: Tridoshic and provides nourishing healthy fats.
- Cinnamon: Adds warmth, helping to balance Kapha and Vata doshas.

Cucumber Raita

A cooling and refreshing yogurt-based side dish or dip, perfect for balancing Pitta dosha and soothing the digestive system.

Prep: 10 mins | Tota: 10 mins | Serves: 2

Ingredients

- 1 cup plain whole-milk yogurt (organic, if possible)
- 1 cucumber, peeled, seeded, and finely diced or grated
- 1/4 cup chopped fresh cilantro or mint
- 1 tablespoon freshly squeezed lime juice
- 1/4 teaspoon ground cumin
- 1/4 teaspoon ground coriander
- Pinch of black pepper
- Pinch of Himalayan pink salt or rock salt (to taste)

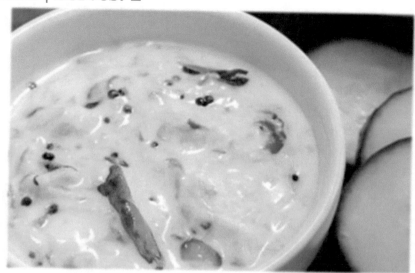

Preparation

1. In a medium bowl, combine the yogurt, cucumber, cilantro or mint, lime juice, cumin, coriander, black pepper, and salt.
2. Stir well to combine all the ingredients.
3. Put in a refrigerator and allow to chill for a minimum of 30 minutes to let the flavors meld.
4. Serve chilled as a side dish or dip with vegetables, crackers, or your favorite Ayurvedic meal.

Nutrition

Calories: 80 | Protein: 4g | Fat: 5g | Carbs: 5g | Fiber: 1g

Ayurvedic Considerations

- Doshas: Balancing for Pitta, can be slightly aggravating for Vata and Kapha in excess.
- Benefits: Cooling, hydrating, aids digestion, balances Pitta, promotes gut health.
- Tips: Use fresh, organic ingredients whenever possible. Adjust spices to your taste and dosha type.

Hard-Boiled Eggs with Turmeric

Enjoy a protein-packed snack that's perfect for balancing Vata dosha. The anti-inflammatory benefits of turmeric and the digestive boost from black pepper make this a nutritious and flavorful choice.

Prep: 2 mins | Cook: 12 mins | Total: 14 mins | Serves: 2

Ingredients

- 2 eggs
- 1/4 teaspoon turmeric powder
- 1/8 teaspoon black pepper powder
- Pinch of sea salt (optional)

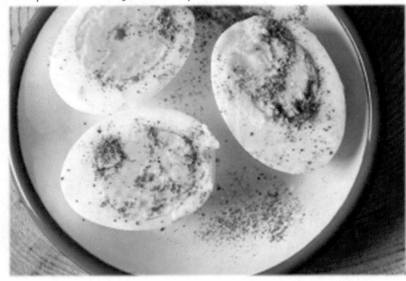

Preparation

1. Boil Eggs: Place the eggs in a saucepan, covering them with cold water.
2. Simmer: Bring the water to a boil, then lower the heat and simmer for 10-12 minutes.
3. Cool Eggs: Drain the hot water and cool the eggs immediately under cold running water.
4. Peel and Season: Peel the eggs and roll them gently in a mixture of turmeric powder, black pepper powder, and a pinch of salt.

Nutrition

Calories: 78 | Protein: 6g | Fat: 5g | Carbs: 1g

Ayurvedic Considerations

Spiced Carrot Sticks with Hummus

Carrots offer a rich source of beta-carotene and fiber, roasted with cumin and coriander for added warmth, while hummus made from chickpeas and tahini delivers protein and healthy fats.

Prep: 10 mins | Cook: 20 mins | Total: 30 mins | Serves: 2

Ingredients

For the Carrots

- 4-5 medium carrots, peeled and cut into sticks
- 1 tablespoon ghee
- 1 teaspoon cumin seeds
- 1/2 teaspoon coriander powder
- 1/4 teaspoon turmeric powder
- Salt, to taste

For the Hummus

- 1 cup cooked chickpeas
- 1/4 cup tahini
- 2 tablespoons lemon juice
- 1 tablespoon olive oil
- 1 clove garlic, minced
- Salt, to taste

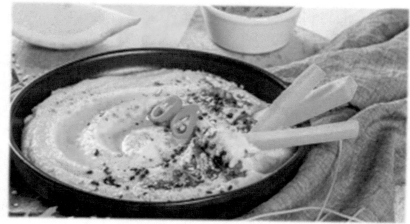

Preparation

1. Roast the Carrots: Preheat your oven to 400°F (200°C). Toss the carrot sticks with ghee, cumin seeds, coriander powder, turmeric powder, and salt. Spread them out on a baking sheet and roast for 20 minutes, or until tender and lightly caramelized.
2. Make the Hummus: In a food processor, combine the chickpeas, tahini, lemon juice, olive oil, garlic, and salt. Blend until smooth and creamy, adding water as needed to reach your preferred consistency.
3. Serve: Arrange the roasted carrot sticks on a platter and serve with the hummus.

Nutrition

Calories: 150 | Protein: 5g | Fat: 8g | Carbs: 15g | Fiber: 5g

Ayurvedic Considerations

- Tridoshic Snack: This snack is suitable for all three doshas (Vata, Pitta, and Kapha).
- Balancing Vata: The warming spices help balance Vata.
- Cooling Pitta: The lemon in the hummus offers cooling properties.
- Digestive Health: High fiber content aids in digestion and elimination

Baked Kale Chips

A light, crispy, and flavorful snack that's packed with nutrients and dosha-balancing properties.

Prep: 10 mins | Cook: 15 mins | Total: 25 mins | Serves: 4

Ingredients

- 1 large bunch of kale, stems removed and leaves torn into bite-sized pieces
- One (1) tbsp. olive oil or coconut oil
- 1/2 teaspoon cumin powder
- 1/4 teaspoon turmeric powder
- 1/4 teaspoon black pepper
- Pinch of Himalayan salt

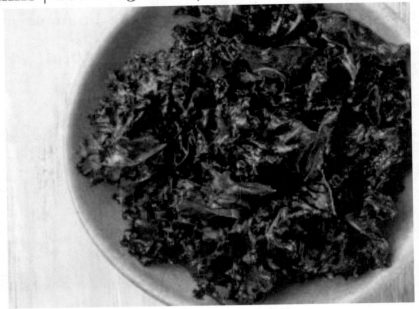

Preparation

1. To begin, first preheat your oven to 300°F (150°C).
2. Wash and thoroughly dry the kale leaves.
3. In a large bowl, toss the kale with the oil and spices until evenly coated.
4. Arrange the kale in a single layer on a baking sheet you already lined with parchment paper.
5. Bake for 10-15 minutes, or until the edges are brown and crispy, but not burnt.
6. Let cool completely before serving.

Nutrition

Calories: 70 | Fat: 5g | Carbs: 6g | Protein: 3g | Fiber: 2g

Ayurvedic Considerations

- Vata: The warming spices and grounding oil make this snack Vata-pacifying.
- Pitta: The bitterness of kale helps balance Pitta, while the cooling spices like coriander and cumin help to cool excess heat.
- Kapha: Kale is naturally drying and light, making it a good choice for Kapha. Use coconut oil for added Kapha-pacifying properties.

Banana Nice Cream

A naturally sweet, cooling, and creamy treat perfect for balancing Pitta and satisfying sweet cravings.

Prep: 5 mins | Total: 5 mins | Serves: 1

Ingredients

- 2 ripe bananas, frozen and sliced
- 1/4 cup coconut milk (or almond milk)
- 1/4 teaspoon cardamom powder
- Pinch of saffron threads (optional)

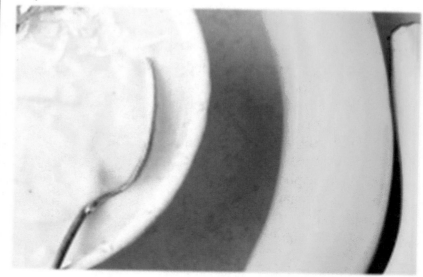

Preparation

1. Freeze ripe banana slices for at least 4 hours.
2. Place frozen banana slices, coconut milk, cardamom powder, and saffron (if using) in a blender or food processor.
3. Blend until smooth and creamy.
4. For a soft-serve consistency, serve right away; for a firmer texture, freeze.

Nutrition

Calories: 150 | Fat: 1g | Carbs: 35g | Fiber: 4g | Protein: 2g

Ayurvedic Considerations

1. Bananas are considered tridoshic, meaning they balance all three doshas in moderation. However, due to their sweetness and cooling nature, they are particularly beneficial for Pitta dosha.
2. Saffron is a luxurious spice that has a calming effect on the mind and body.

Guacamole with Veggie Sticks

This creamy and refreshing Ayurvedic guacamole is a perfect snack or appetizer. It's packed with healthy fats, fiber, and flavor, making it a satisfying and nourishing option for all doshas.

Prep: 10 mins | Total: 8-10 mins | Serves: 2

Ingredients

- 2 ripe avocados
- 1/4 cup finely chopped red onion
- 1/4 cup finely chopped cilantro
- 1/4 cup finely chopped tomatoes
- 1 tablespoon lime juice
- 1/2 teaspoon cumin powder
- 1/4 teaspoon coriander powder
- Pinch of Himalayan salt
- Pinch of black pepper
- Assorted raw vegetables for dipping (carrots, cucumbers, celery, bell peppers)

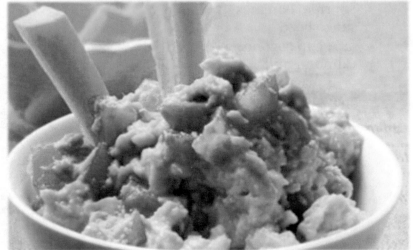

Preparation

1. Get a medium bowl, cut the avocado open and mash your avocados with a fork until smooth.
2. Add the red onion, cilantro, tomatoes, lime juice, cumin, coriander, salt, and pepper.
3. Mix well to combine.
4. Serve with assorted raw vegetables for dipping.

Nutrition

Calories: 150 | Fat: 14g | Carbs: 6g | Protein: 2g | Fiber: 5g

Ayurvedic Considerations

- Vata: This dish is grounding and nourishing for Vata due to the healthy fats and creamy texture of the avocados.
- Pitta: The cooling properties of cilantro and lime juice help balance Pitta.
- Kapha: The spices and vegetables help to reduce Kapha's heaviness.

DESSERTS

DEAR READER

Your journey through the flavors and wisdom of Ayurveda has been a true inspiration to us. As you continue to explore the recipes and practices within these pages, we invite you to share your experience with us. Your feedback is invaluable in helping us create resources that truly nourish and empower women on their path to well-being.

We'd be delighted if you could take a moment to leave an honest review of this cookbook. Your insights, whether they be about a favorite recipe, a transformative ritual, or a newfound understanding of Ayurvedic principles, will help guide other women on their own journeys. By sharing your thoughts, you become a part of our growing community of women supporting and inspiring each other. We are deeply grateful for your support and look forward to hearing your voice.

Cardamom and Saffron Rice Pudding

It's naturally sweet and easy to digest, making it a comforting treat for all doshas.

Prep: 10 mins | Cook: 50 mins | Total: 60 mins | Serves: 4

Ingredients

- 1/2 cup basmati rice, rinsed
- 4 cups milk (cow's milk or plant-based milk like almond or coconut)
- A quarter (1/4) cup jaggery or raw sugar (adjust to taste)
- A quarter (1/4) teaspoon cardamom powder
- 2 tablespoons ghee (clarified butter)
- A handful of raisins
- A handful of chopped almonds
- A pinch of saffron strands (optional)
- 1/4 teaspoon ground cinnamon (optional)
- A few crushed pistachios for garnish (optional)

Preparation

1. In a bowl, soak the rinsed rice in water for 30 minutes. Drain and set aside.
2. In a saucepan, combine the soaked rice and milk. Bring to a boil, then reduce heat and simmer, stirring occasionally, for about 30-35 minutes, or until the rice is soft and the milk has thickened.
3. Add the jaggery or raw sugar and stir until it dissolves completely.
4. Add the cardamom powder, raisins, chopped almonds, saffron strands (if using), and ground cinnamon (if using). Ensure to stir well and allow it simmer for another 5-10 mins.
5. At this time, you can taste the kheer and adjust to suit your taste by adding more jaggery or sugar if necessary.
6. Once the rice pudding reaches your desired doneness and the rice is fully cooked, turn off the heat. Let the kheer cool for some minutes. This allows it to thicken further as it cools down. Serve warm or chilled, garnished with crushed pistachios if desired.

Nutrition

Calories: 290 | kcal | Carbs: 33g | Protein: 7g | Fat: 14g

Ayurvedic Considerations

- Vata: This kheer is naturally sweet and grounding, making it balancing for Vata. The addition of warming spices like cardamom and cinnamon further pacifies Vata.
- Pitta: For Pitta individuals, use less jaggery or sugar and consider using coconut milk instead of cow's milk to make it more cooling.
- Kapha: For Kapha individuals, use less rice and more milk to make a thinner kheer. Avoid using sugar and limit the amount of ghee.

Spiced Baked Apples with Nuts and Raisins

A warm, comforting Ayurvedic dessert that's perfect for fall and winter. Apples are baked with warming spices, ghee, nuts, and raisins, creating a naturally sweet and satisfying treat.

Prep: 10 mins | Cook: 30 mins | Total: 40 mins | Serves: 4

Ingredients

- 4 medium-sized apples (organic, if possible)
- 2 tablespoons ghee (clarified butter)
- 1/4 cup chopped walnuts or pecans
- 1/4 cup raisins
- 1 teaspoon ground cinnamon
- 1/2 teaspoon ground cardamom
- 1/4 teaspoon ground nutmeg
- A pinch of sea salt

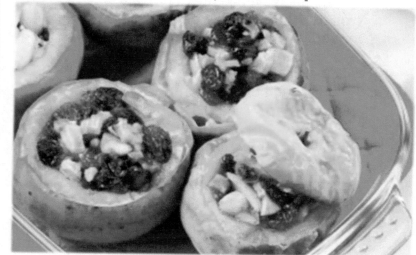

Preparation

1. Preheat oven to 350°F (175°C).
2. Wash and core the apples, leaving a small well in the center of each.
3. In a small bowl, combine the ghee, nuts, raisins, cinnamon, cardamom, nutmeg, and salt.
4. Fill each apple with the spice and nut mixture.
5. Place the apples in a baking dish and bake for 25-30 minutes, or until the apples are tender when pierced with a fork.
6. Serve warm with a dollop of coconut yogurt or whipped cream (optional).

Nutrition

Calories: 200 | Carbs: 28g | Fiber: 5g | Protein: 2g | Fat: 11g

Ayurvedic Considerations

- Apples are considered tridoshic, meaning they are balancing for all three doshas (Vata, Pitta, and Kapha).
- Ghee is a nourishing fat that supports digestion and provides essential vitamins.
- Warming spices like cinnamon, cardamom, and nutmeg help to balance Vata and Kapha dosha.
- Nuts and raisins provide healthy fats, fiber, and protein.

Mango Lassi

A refreshing and cooling Ayurvedic drink, perfect for balancing Pitta dosha during hot weather or after a spicy meal.

Prep: 5 mins | Total: 5 mins | Serves: 2

Ingredients

- 1 ripe mango, peeled and chopped
- 1 cup plain whole milk yogurt (homemade or organic)
- 1/2 cup milk (dairy or plant-based)
- 1/4 teaspoon cardamom powder
- A sprinkle of saffron threads (optional for garnish).
- 1-2 teaspoons honey or jaggery (optional, to taste)

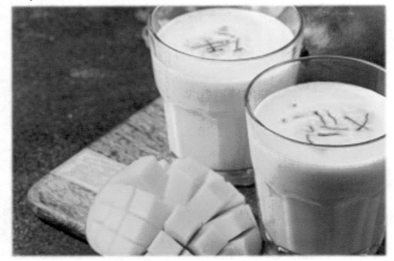

Preparation

1. Combine all ingredients in a blender.
2. Blend until smooth and creamy.
3. Taste and adjust sweetness if needed.
4. Pour into your glasses and top with saffron threads.

Nutrition

Calories: 180 | Protein: 8g | Carbs: 21g | Fat:8g | Fiber: 3g

Ayurvedic Considerations

- Mango is considered a tridoshic fruit, meaning it is generally balancing for all three doshas. However, its sweetness can increase Kapha, so use it in moderation if you have a Kapha imbalance.
- Yogurt is cooling and nourishing, making it ideal for Pitta dosha. It also contains probiotics, which support digestion and gut health.
- Cardamom is a digestive aid that helps reduce bloating and gas. It also has a warming effect that balances Vata dosha.
- Honey or jaggery are natural sweeteners that are considered more balancing in Ayurveda than refined sugar. However, still used them in moderation.

Carrot Halwa

Carrot Halwa, also known as Gajar Ka Halwa, is a beloved Indian dessert that embodies the principles of Ayurveda. It's a perfect way to satisfy your sweet tooth while providing your body with essential nutrients and balancing the doshas.

Pre: 15 mins | Cook: 60 mins | Total: 1 hr. 15 mins | Serves: 4-6

Ingredients

- 1 kg carrots, washed, peeled, and grated
- 500 ml full-fat milk (cow's milk or plant-based milk like almond or cashew milk)
- 1/4 cup ghee (clarified butter) or coconut oil
- 1/4 cup jaggery powder or coconut sugar
- 1 teaspoon cardamom powder
- Pinch of saffron strands (optional)
- 2 tablespoons chopped almonds and pistachios

Preparation

1. In a heavy-bottomed pan, heat the ghee or coconut oil over medium heat. Add the grated carrots and sauté for 5-7 minutes, stirring occasionally, until they soften and release their natural sweetness.

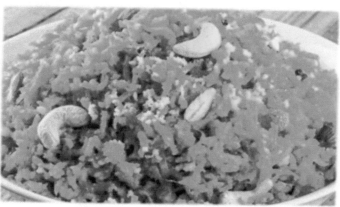

2. Add the milk, jaggery or coconut sugar, and saffron (if using) to the pan. Generously Mix thoroughly and bring to a simmer.
3. Reduce the heat to low and cook for 45-60 minutes, stirring regularly, until the milk is absorbed and the halwa thickens. The halwa should have a creamy texture and a rich orange color.
4. Stir in the cardamom powder and chopped nuts. Gently simmer for additional 2-3 mins until fragrant.
5. Remove from heat and serve warm.

Nutrition

Calories: 300 | Carbs: 30g | Protein: 7g | Fat: 20g

Ayurvedic Considerations

- This recipe is suitable for all doshas in moderation.
- The sweetness from the jaggery or coconut sugar is balanced by the carrots' natural sweetness.
- Ghee or coconut oil provides healthy fats and aids digestion.
- Cardamom, saffron, and nuts offer additional warmth and nourishment.

Coconut Ladoo

These delightful Coconut Ladoos are a perfect Ayurvedic treat, balancing all three doshas with their sweet, warming, and grounding properties.

Prep: 10 mins | Total: 10 mins | Serves: 12 ladoos

Ingredients

- 1 cup shredded unsweetened coconut
- 1/2 cup pitted dates, soaked in warm water for 10 minutes
- 1/4 cup chopped nuts (almonds, cashews, or walnuts)
- 2 tablespoons ghee (clarified butter)
- 1/4 teaspoon cardamom powder
- Pinch of saffron strands (optional)

Tips

- For a richer flavor, you can lightly toast the shredded coconut before using it.
- If the mixture is too dry, add a tablespoon or two of warm water.
- If the mixture is not thick enough, add a bit more shredded coconut.
- Feel free to experiment with different nuts and seeds, such as pistachios, pumpkin seeds, or sunflower seeds.
- You can also add a pinch of other warming spices like nutmeg or ginger for additional flavor and therapeutic benefits

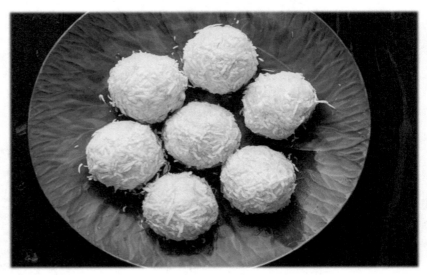

Preparation

1. Drain the soaked dates and discard the water.
2. In a food processor, combine the shredded coconut, dates, nuts, ghee, cardamom powder, and saffron (if using).
3. Pulse the ingredients until they come together to form a sticky dough.
4. Roll the dough into small balls (about 1 inch in diameter) using your hands.
5. Store the ladoos in an airtight container at room temperature for up to a week, or in the refrigerator for longer shelf life.

Nutrition

Calories: 100 | Protein: 2g | Fat: 6g | Carbs: 8g | Fiber: 2g

Spiced Poached Pears

A comforting and fragrant Ayurvedic dessert featuring pears gently cooked in a spiced syrup, perfect for balancing Vata and Pitta doshas. This recipe is naturally sweet, warming, and easy to digest.

Prep: 5 mins | Cook: 20 mins | Total: 25 mins | Serves: 4

Ingredients

- 4 ripe but firm pears (Bosc or Anjou work well)
- 4 cups water
- 1/4 cup raw honey or maple syrup
- 2-inch piece of fresh ginger, thinly sliced
- 4 cardamom pods, lightly crushed
- 1 cinnamon stick
- Pinch of saffron threads (optional)

Preparation

1. Get your ready by peeling and cutting them in half lengthwise. remove the core and seeds using spoon or a melon baller if you have one.
2. Combine the water, honey (or maple syrup), ginger, cardamom, cinnamon, and saffron (if using) in a saucepan.
3. Heat the mixture bring to a simmer over medium heat.
4. Add the pears to the saucepan, making sure they are submerged in the liquid.
5. Low the heat and cover the mixture. Simmer again for additional 15-20 mins, or until the pears are tender when pierced with a fork.
6. Then, gently remove the pears from the saucepan and put them in a serving bowl.
7. Increase the heat to medium and simmer the liquid for a few more minutes, or until it has reduced and thickened slightly.
8. Drizzle the spiced syrup over the pears and serve warm or chilled.

Nutrition

Calories: 150 | Carbs: 35g | Protein: 1g | Fat: 1g | Fiber: 5g

Ayurvedic Considerations

- Vata Dosha: This recipe is calming and grounding for Vata due to the cooked fruit, sweet taste, and warming spices.
- Pitta Dosha: The sweetness of the pears and honey balances Pitta, while the cooling spices like cardamom and cinnamon help to pacify any excess heat.
- Kapha Dosha: Kapha individuals may want to use less sweetener and add a pinch of black pepper to the poaching liquid for a more stimulating effect.

Ayurvedic Date and Nut Truffles

These bite-sized delights are a perfect Ayurvedic treat, balancing sweetness with the grounding qualities of nuts and spices. They are naturally sweet, packed with fiber and healthy fats, and require no cooking.

Prep: 15 mins | Total: 15 mins | Serves: 12 truffles

Ingredients

- 1 cup pitted Medjool date
- 1/2 cup raw almonds
- 1/4 cup shredded coconut
- 1 tablespoon coconut oil, melted
- 1/2 teaspoon ground cardamom
- Pinch of sea salt

Ayurvedic Considerations

- Dates provide natural sweetness and are considered tridoshic (balancing for all three doshas).
- For a Vata-balancing variation, add a pinch of warming spices like ginger or nutmeg.
- For a Pitta-balancing variation, reduce the amount of cardamom or omit it altogether.
- To make these truffles more Kapha-balancing, use less coconut and dates, and add a pinch of black pepper.

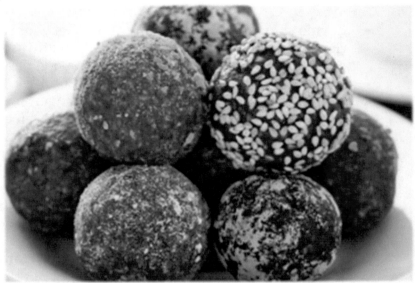

Preparation

1. Gather the dates and almond, combine them In a food processor. Pulse until a sticky dough forms.
2. Add the coconut, coconut oil, cardamom, and salt. Pulse again until well combined.
3. Roll the mixture into small balls (about 1 tablespoon each).
4. If desired, roll the truffles in additional shredded coconut.
5. For a delightful taste, refrigerate for at least 30 mins to firm up before serving.

Nutrition

Calories: 90 | Protein: 2g | Fat: 5g | Carbs: 10g | Fiber: 2g

Ayurvedic Sweet Potato Pudding

This warm and comforting pudding is a nourishing and satisfying dessert that's perfect for balancing Vata dosha. The natural sweetness of sweet potatoes combined with warming spices creates a delightful treat that's both delicious and healthy.

Prep: 10 mins | Cook: 30 mins | Total: 40 mins | Serves: 4

Ingredients

- 2 large sweet potatoes, peeled and cubed
- 1 cup coconut milk
- 1/4 cup jaggery or maple syrup (adjust to taste)
- 1 teaspoon ground cinnamon
- 1/2 teaspoon ground cardamom
- 1/4 teaspoon ground nutmeg
- Pinch of sea salt

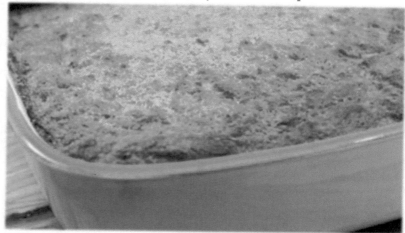

Ayurvedic Considerations

- Vata-Balancing: The sweet and warming nature of sweet potatoes and spices helps to balance Vata dosha.
- Nourishing: Sweet potatoes are a good source of fiber, vitamin A, and vitamin C, while coconut milk provides healthy fats.
- Easy to Digest: The simple ingredients and cooking method make this pudding easy to digest.

Preparation

Steam the sweet potatoes until tender.

1. Mash the sweet potatoes thoroughly.
2. In a saucepan, combine the mashed sweet potatoes, coconut milk, jaggery or maple syrup, cinnamon, cardamom, nutmeg, and salt.
3. Cook over low heat, stirring constantly, until the mixture thickens and becomes pudding-like.
4. For a maximum treat serve warm, topped with a sprinkle of cinnamon.

Nutrition

Calories: 200 | Fat: 10g | Carbs: 30g | Protein: 3g | Fiber: 4g

Spiced Fruit Compote

Prep: 10 mins | Cook: 25 mins | Total: 35 mins | Serves: 4

Ingredients

- 2 cups chopped apples (preferably a sweet variety)
- 1 cup chopped pears
- 1/2 cup chopped plums or peaches (seasonal)
- 1/4 cup raisins or chopped dates
- 1/4 cup water
- 1/2 teaspoon ground cinnamon
- 1/4 teaspoon ground cardamom
- 1/8 teaspoon ground cloves
- Pinch of nutmeg (optional)
- 1 tablespoon ghee (optional, for added richness)

Ayurvedic Considerations

- This recipe is naturally sweet and warming, making it ideal for balancing Vata dosha.
- The spices used in this recipe aid digestion and have warming properties.
- Ghee is considered a nourishing and healing fat in Ayurveda.
- Adjust the amount of sweetener to your taste and dosha type.

Preparation

1. In a saucepan, combine the chopped fruits, raisins or dates, and water.
2. Add the cinnamon, cardamom, cloves, and nutmeg (if using).

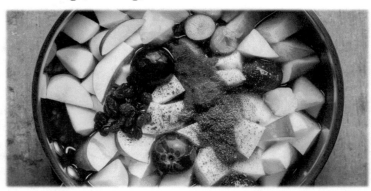

3. If desired, add ghee for a richer flavor and additional nourishment.
4. Over medium heat, bring the mixture to a moderate simmer.
5. Reduce heat to low, cover, and cook for 20-25 minutes, or until the fruits are tender and the liquid has thickened slightly.
6. Remove from heat and allow it cool for a few minutes before serving.
7. Optional Additions
8. A sprinkle of chopped nuts, such as almonds or walnuts, for added crunch and protein.
9. A dollop of coconut yogurt or whipped coconut cream for extra richness.
10. A drizzle of maple syrup or honey for additional sweetness, if desired.

Nutrition

Calories: 145 | Carbs: 20g | Fiber: 5g | Sugar: 15g | Protein: 2g

Spiced Pear Crumble

This warm and comforting dessert is perfect for balancing Vata dosha during colder months. Sweet pears, warming spices, and a crunchy oat topping make it a delightful treat.

Prep: 15 mins | Cook: 30 mins | Total: 45 mins | Serves: 4

Ingredients

Filling

- 4 ripe but firm pears, peeled, cored, and sliced
- 1 tablespoon ghee (clarified butter)
- 1 teaspoon ground cinnamon
- Half (1/2) teaspoon ground cardamom
- A quarter (1/4) teaspoon ground nutmeg
- Pinch of ground cloves
- 2 tablespoons maple syrup (or jaggery powder)

Crumble Topping

- Half (1/2) cup rolled oats
- Half (1/2) cup chopped nuts (almonds, walnuts, or pecans)
- 2 tablespoons ghee
- 2 tablespoons maple syrup (or jaggery powder)

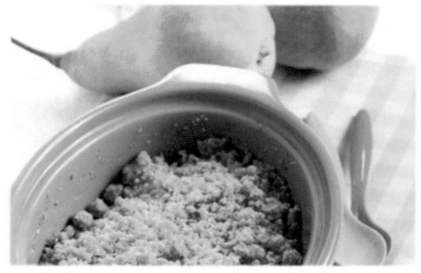

Preparation

1. To begin, first preheat your oven to 375°F (190°C).
2. In a bowl, combine the sliced pears, ghee, cinnamon, cardamom, nutmeg, cloves, and maple syrup. Toss to coat evenly.
3. In a separate bowl, mix the oats, chopped nuts, ghee, and maple syrup until well combined.
4. Gently arrange the pear mixture evenly in a baking dish. Crumble the oat mixture over the pears.
5. Bake for 30 minutes, or until the pears are tender and the crumble is golden brown.
6. Serve warm with a dollop of coconut yogurt or whipped coconut cream.

Nutrition

Calories: 250 | Fat: 15g | Carbs: 28g | Fiber: 5g | Protein: 4g

Ayurvedic Considerations

- This recipe is balancing for Vata dosha due to the use of warming spices, ghee, and cooked fruit.
- Adjust the spices to suit your individual taste and dosha balance.
- Use seasonal pears for optimal flavor and nutrition.
- For a Pitta-pacifying version, reduce or omit the warming spices like cloves and ginger.

Coconut Milk Panna Cotta with Mango Coulis

Prep: 15 mins | Cook: 5 mins | Total: 4 hrs. 20 mins | Serves: 4

Ingredients

- 1 (14-ounce) can full-fat coconut milk
- 1/4 cup maple syrup
- 1/2 teaspoon ground cardamom
- 1 tablespoon agar agar flakes or powder
- 1 ripe mango, peeled and chopped
- 1 tablespoon lime juice

Ayurvedic Considerations

- o Vata: The warming spices and grounding coconut milk help balance Vata.
- o Pitta: The sweetness of the mango and coconut milk helps pacify Pitta, while the lime juice adds a cooling element.
- o Kapha: The light and refreshing nature of the mango coulis helps balance Kapha. The small portion size is also suitable for Kapha

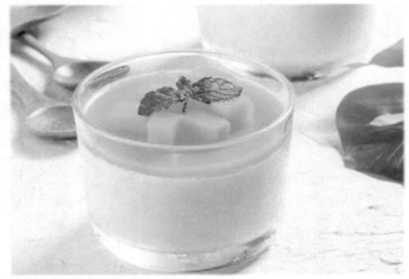

Preparation

1. In a small saucepan, combine agar agar with 2 tablespoons of water. Allow to rest for 5 minutes so as to bloom.
2. In a separate saucepan, combine coconut milk, maple syrup, and cardamom. Heat untin simmering over medium heat.
3. Whisk in the bloomed agar agar mixture. Continue to simmer for 2-3 minutes, or until the agar agar is fully dissolved.
4. Pour the mixture into four ramekins or small bowls. Refrigerate them for at least four (4) so as to set.
5. While the panna cotta is chilling, add the mango and lime juice and blend until smooth. If desired, strain through a fine-mesh sieve to remove any fibers.
6. Once the panna cotta is set, top each serving with a generous spoonful of mango coulis. Garnish with fresh mint leaves or a sprinkle of shredded coconut, if desired.

Nutrition

Calories: 250 | Fat: 18g | Carbs: 20g | Protein: 2g

Spiced Ayurvedic Banana Bread

Prep: 15 mins | Cook: 50 mins | Total: 1 hr. | Serves: 8 slices

Ingredients

- 3 ripe bananas, mashed
- 1/4 cup ghee or coconut oil, melted
- 1/4 cup honey or maple syrup
- 2 eggs
- 1 teaspoon vanilla extract
- 1 1/2 cups almond flour
- 1/2 teaspoon baking soda
- 1/2 teaspoon ground cinnamon
- 1/4 teaspoon ground cardamom
- 1/4 teaspoon salt
- Optional: Chopped nuts or seeds for topping

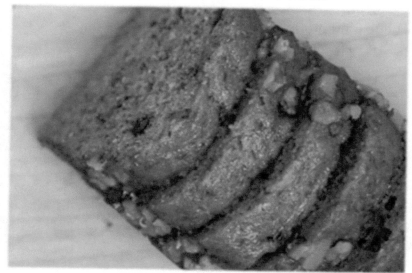

Preparation

1. To start, first preheat your oven to 350°F (175°C) and then grease your loaf pan.
2. Get a large bowl, whisk together eggs, ghee, mashed bananas, honey, and vanilla extract until well combined.
3. In another bowl, mix together baking soda, cardamom, almond flour, cinnamon, and salt.
4. Mix in the dry ingredients to the wet ingredients and vigorously mix until just well combined. Do not overmix.
5. Add in chopped nuts or seeds but this is optional
6. Pour batter into the prepared loaf pan and bake for 45-50 minutes, or until a toothpick inserted into the center comes out clean.
7. When done, allow it cool in the pan for 10 mins and then transfer to a wire rack to cool completely.

Nutrition

Calories: 180 | Fat: 12g | Carbs: 15g | Protein: 4g | Fiber: 2g

Almond Flour Cardamom Cookies

Prep: 10 mins | Cook: 15 mins | Total: 25 mins | Serves: 12 cookies

Ingredients

1 cup almond flour

- 1/4 cup coconut oil, melted
- 1/4 cup maple syrup or honey
- 1/4 teaspoon ground cardamom
- 1/4 teaspoon vanilla extract
- Pinch of sea salt

Ayurvedic Considerations

- o Vata: The warming spices and grounding almond flour help to balance Vata.
- o Pitta: The sweetness of maple syrup or honey is cooling and balancing for Pitta.
- o Kapha: The small portion size and use of almond flour instead of wheat flour make these cookies lighter and easier to digest for Kapha.

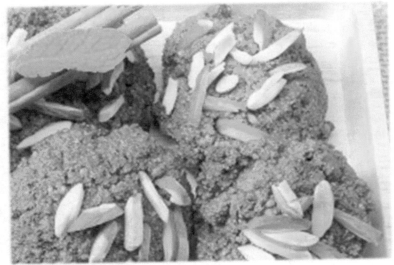

Preparation

1. To start, first preheat your oven to 350°F (175°C) and then line your baking sheet with parchment paper.
2. In a medium bowl, combine almond flour, coconut oil, maple syrup or honey, cardamom, vanilla extract, and salt. Mix until a dough forms.
3. Roll dough into 12 small balls. Place on the prepared baking sheet and flatten slightly with your fingers.
4. Bake for 12-15 minutes while checking at intervals, or until the dough is golden brown around the edges.
5. Set and allow it cool completely on the baking sheet before serving.

Nutrition

Calories: 100 | Fat: 8g | Carbs: 6g | Protein: 3g

Quinoa and Apple Crumble

A warm and comforting dessert that balances the doshas with whole grains, fruit, and warming spices.

Prep: 10 mins | Cook: 30 mins | Total: 40 mins | Serves: 4

Ingredients

Filling

- 1 cup cooked quinoa
- 2 apples, peeled, cored, and diced
- 1/4 cup raisins (soaked in warm water for 10 minutes and drained)
- 1/4 cup chopped walnuts
- 1/4 cup chopped dates
- 1/2 teaspoon ground cinnamon
- 1/4 teaspoon ground cardamom
- Pinch of ground nutmeg

Crumble Topping

- 1/2 cup rolled oats
- 1/4 cup almond flour
- 1/4 cup chopped pecans or almonds
- 2 tablespoons ghee or coconut oil, melted
- 2 tablespoons maple syrup or honey

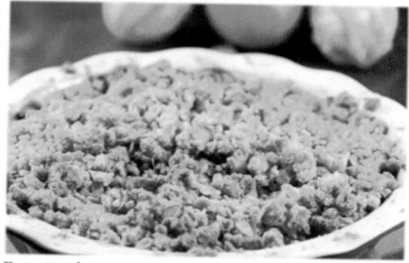

Preparation

1. Preheat oven to 350°F (175°C).
2. In a bowl, combine cooked quinoa, apples, raisins, walnuts, dates, cinnamon, cardamom, and nutmeg.
3. In a separate bowl, combine rolled oats, almond flour, pecans, melted ghee, and maple syrup. Mix until well combined and crumbly.
4. In a baking dish, spread the quinoa and apple mixture evenly.
5. Crumble the topping mixture over the fruit mixture.
6. Bake for 25-30 minutes, or until the topping is golden brown and the fruit is tender.
7. Serve warm with a dollop of coconut yogurt or whipped cream (optional).

Nutrition

Calories: 350 | Protein: 8g | Fat: 18g | Carbs: 35g | Fiber: 7g | Sugar: 15g

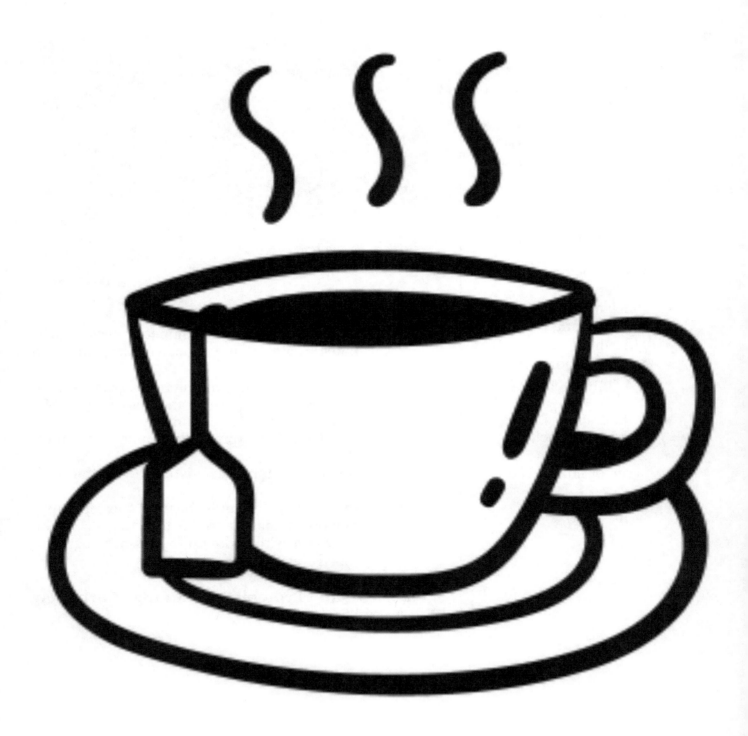

Ginger Lemon Tea

This warming and invigorating tea combines the digestive power of ginger with the cleansing properties of lemon, making it a perfect Ayurvedic beverage to sip throughout the day.

Prep: 5 mins | Cook: 10-12 mins | Total: 15-17 mins | Serves: 1

Ingredients

- One (1) inch piece peeled and thinly sliced fresh ginger
- 1/2 lemon, juiced
- 1 teaspoon raw honey (optional)
- 1 cup filtered water

Ayurvedic Considerations

- Doshas: Balancing for all doshas, especially Vata and Kapha.
- Benefits: Aids digestion, boosts immunity, relieves nausea, and warms the body.

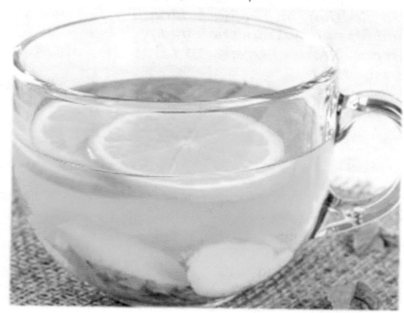

Preparation

1. In a small saucepan, combine the ginger slices and water.
2. Heat the mixture until starts to boil, then low the heat and simmer for 10 minutes.
3. Take the mixture of the heat and add 1/2 lemon juice.
4. Using a fine-mesh sieve and strain the mixture into a cup and add honey if desired.
5. Sip warm and enjoy!

Nutrition

Calories: 11.2 | Carbs: 3.5g | Protein: 0g | Fat: 1g

CCF Tea (Cumin, Coriander, Fennel)

This simple yet potent tea, made with cumin, coriander, and fennel seeds, is a staple in Ayurvedic kitchens. It gently ignites your digestive fire (agni), aids in detoxification, and reduces bloating and gas. Enjoy it after meals or as a daily ritual for optimal digestion and well-being.

Prep: 5 mins | Cook: 10 mins | Total: 15 mins | Serves: 1

Ingredients

- 1 teaspoon cumin seeds
- 1 teaspoon coriander seeds
- 1 teaspoon fennel seeds
- 2 cups water

Ayurvedic Considerations

- Add a pinch of ginger powder for extra warmth and digestive support.
- To sweeten add a teaspoon of raw honey or maple syrup as desired.
- According to Ayurveda, this tea is considered tridoshic, meaning it is suitable for all three doshas (Vata, Pitta, and Kapha).
- Enjoy a cup of CCF tea after meals to aid digestion or sip throughout the day for a gentle detox.
- If you experience any discomfort, reduce the amount of spice.

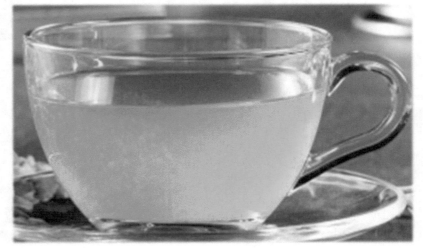

Preparation

1. In a small saucepan, combine the cumin, coriander, and fennel seeds.
2. Dry roast the seeds over low heat for 1-2 minutes until fragrant, stirring constantly to prevent burning.
3. Add the 2 cups of water to the saucepan and bring to a boil.
4. Low the heat, cover the saucepan, and simmer again for 10 minutes.
5. Using a clean fine-mesh sieve strain the tea into a cup.
6. Sip slowly and enjoy!

Nutrition

Calories: 5 | Fat: 0g | Carbs: 1g | Protein: 0g

Tulsi Tea (Holy Basil Tea)

Tulsi, or holy basil, is revered in Ayurveda for its adaptogenic and stress-reducing properties. This simple tea is both calming and refreshing, making it a perfect way to unwind and nourish your body.

Prep: 2-5mins | Cook: 5 mins | Total: 7-10 mins | Serves: 1

Ingredients

- 10-15 fresh tulsi leaves (or 2 teaspoons dried tulsi)
- 1 1/2 cups water

Ayurvedic Tips

- Tulsi tea is balancing for all three doshas, but particularly beneficial for Vata and Pitta.
- Drink tulsi tea regularly to help manage stress, boost immunity, and promote overall well-being.
- For a stronger brew, use more tulsi leaves or simmer for a longer period.
- To enhance the flavor and therapeutic benefits, combine tulsi with other herbs like ginger, mint, or chamomile.

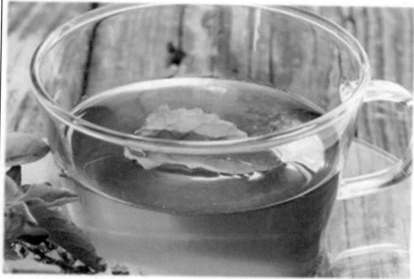

Preparation

1. Rinse the fresh tulsi leaves thoroughly.
2. Add the leaves to a saucepan with the water.
3. Gently heat and bring to a boil, then reduce heat and simmer for 5 minutes.
4. Using a fine-mesh sieve strain the tea into a cup and enjoy warm.
5. Optional Additions
6. Add a slice of fresh ginger for extra warmth and digestive support.
7. Sweeten with a teaspoon of raw honey or a few drops of stevia.

Nutrition

Calories: 2 | Carbs: 0g | Protein: 0g | Fat: 0g

Rose and Cardamom Iced Tea

A delicate and refreshing Ayurvedic iced tea that combines the floral notes of rose with the warming spice of cardamom. This caffeine-free drink is naturally sweet and cooling, making it perfect for hot summer days or as a balancing beverage for Pitta dosha.

Prep: 5 mins | Cook: 10 mins | Total: 15 mins | Serves: 4

Ingredients

- 4 cups filtered water
- 1 tablespoon dried rose petals (ensure they are food-grade)
- 8-10 green cardamom pods, lightly crushed
- Honey or maple syrup to taste (optional)
- Fresh rose petals for garnish (optional)

Ayurvedic Considerations

- Rose is cooling and calming, making it beneficial for balancing Pitta dosha.
- Cardamom is warming and aids digestion, making it beneficial for Vata and Kapha doshas.
- Honey or maple syrup can be added for a touch of sweetness, but use them sparingly as excessive sweet taste can increase Kapha.

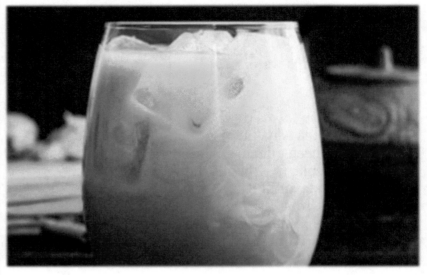

Preparation

1. Add the water to a saucepan, and bring to a boil.
2. Add rose petals and cardamom pods.
3. Next, lower the heat, cover, and simmer for 10 minutes.
4. Remove from heat and let steep for at least 2 hours, or preferably overnight, in the refrigerator.
5. Strain the tea into a pitcher.
6. Add the sweetener (honey or maple syrup) to taste, if desired.
7. Serve chilled, garnished with fresh rose petals, if using.

Nutrition

Calories: 10 | Carbs: 2g | Protein: 2g | Fat: 4g.

Fennel and Mint Tea

This cooling and refreshing tea is perfect for after meals to aid digestion and freshen breath. Fennel is known for its digestive properties, while mint leaves soothe the stomach and cool the body.

Prep: 5 mins | Cook: 7 mins | Total: 12 mins | Serves: 1

Ingredients

- 1 teaspoon fennel seeds
- 5-6 fresh mint leaves
- 1 cup water

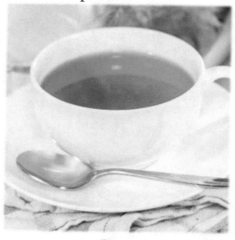

Preparation

1. Heat 1 cup of water in a saucepan until it starts to boil
2. Add the fennel seeds and mint leaves to the boiling water.
3. Then, reduce the heat, cover, and simmer for additional 5-7 mins.
4. Using a fine-mesh sieve, strain the mixture into a cup and enjoy warm.

Nutrition

Calories: 7.5 | Fat: 1g | Cars: 1g | Protein: 0g

Ayurvedic Considerations

- Dosha: This tea is balancing for all doshas, especially Pitta due to its cooling properties.
- Taste: Pungent (fennel), sweet (mint)
- Benefits: Aids digestion, reduces bloating, freshens breath, cools the body.

Coconut Water Refresher

This naturally sweet and refreshing drink is not only hydrating but also helps balance all three doshas, making it a perfect beverage for any time of day.

Prep: 5 mins | Total: 5 mins | Serves: 1

Ingredients

- 1 cup fresh young coconut water (preferably organic)
- 1/2 lime, juiced
- 5-6 fresh mint leaves

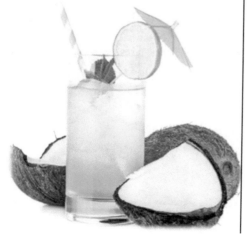

Preparation

1. In a glass, combine the coconut water and lime juice.
2. Gently muddle the mint leaves to release their flavor and aroma.
3. Add the muddled mint leaves to the coconut water mixture.
4. Stir well and enjoy immediately.

Nutrition

Calories: 45 | Carbs: 9g | Sugar: 6g

Ayurvedic Tips

- To make this drink more Vata pacifying, add a pinch of ginger powder or a few slices of fresh ginger.
- For Pitta balancing, you can add a pinch of cumin powder or a few cucumber slices.
- If you have a Kapha imbalance, reduce the amount of coconut water and add a pinch of black pepper.

Ginger Turmeric Iced Tea

This vibrant iced tea is a burst of flavor and a potent dose of anti-inflammatory goodness. Ginger and turmeric, revered in Ayurveda for their warming and healing properties, come together with a touch of honey for sweetness and a squeeze of lemon for brightness. It's the perfect thirst quencher on a hot day or a soothing remedy for aches and pains.

Prep: 5 mins | Cook: 15 mins | Total: 20 mins | Serves: 2

Ingredients

- One (1) inch piece of peeled and thinly sliced fresh ginger
- 1-inch piece fresh peeled and thinly sliced turmeric (or 1 teaspoon ground turmeric)
- 4 cups filtered water
- Honey or maple syrup to taste (optional)
- Juice of 1/2 lemon (optional)

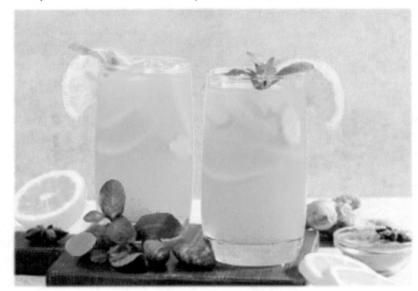

Ayurvedic Considerations

1. Ginger and turmeric are both warming spices that balance Vata and Kapha doshas.
2. Honey is a natural sweetener that is easily digestible.

Preparation

1. Add the ginger, turmeric, and water to a saucepan, combine and bring to a boil.
2. Reduce the heat to low and simmer for additional 15 mins.
3. Take the mixture of the heat source and allow to cool completely.
4. Using a fine-mesh sieve, and strain the tea into a pitcher.
5. Add the (honey or maple syrup) and lemon juice to taste.
6. Put in a refrigerator and chill. Serve over ice.

Nutrition

Calories: 10 | Carbs: 2g | Protein: 0g | Fat: 2.1g

Buttermilk (Masala Chaas)

A refreshing and cooling Ayurvedic drink, perfect for balancing Pitta and soothing digestion.

Prep: 5 mins | Total: 5-7 mins | Serves: 1

Ingredients

- 1/2 cup plain, whole-milk yogurt (organic, if possible)
- 1 cup water (filtered or boiled and cooled)
- 1/4 teaspoon ground cumin
- 1/4 teaspoon ground coriander
- Pinch of pink Himalayan salt
- Few fresh mint leaves, chopped (optional)

Preparation

1. Combine yogurt and water in a blender.
2. Add cumin, coriander, and salt.
3. Blend until frothy and well combined.
4. To serve, pour into a glass cup and top with fresh mint leaves, if desired.

Nutrition

Calories: 80 | Protein: 5g | Fat: 5g | Carbs: 4g

Ayurvedic Tips

- Use room temperature or slightly chilled ingredients for optimal digestion.
- Adjust the amount of spice to your taste preference.
- For Vata imbalance, you can add a pinch of ginger powder.
- For Kapha imbalance, reduce the amount of yogurt and increase the water.

Ginger Beetroot Juice

This vibrant juice is a powerhouse of nutrients and antioxidants, known for its detoxifying and energizing properties.

Prep: 5 mins | Total: 5 mins | Serves: 1

Ingredients

- 1 medium beetroot, peeled and roughly chopped
- 1 medium carrot, peeled and roughly chopped
- 1 medium apple, cored and roughly chopped
- One (1) inch piece freshly peeled and roughly chopped ginger
- Optional: A squeeze of fresh lemon juice (for a touch of brightness)

Preparation

1. Thoroughly wash all ingredients.
2. Pass the beetroot, carrot, apple, and ginger through a juicer.
3. If desired, add a squeeze of lemon juice to taste.
4. Stir well and serve immediately.

Nutrition

Calories: 100 | Carbs: 24g | Fiber: 4g | Sugar: 16g | Protein: 1g | Fat: 2.1g

Ayurvedic Considerations

- Vata: This juice is generally balancing for Vata due to its grounding and warming properties.
- Pitta: Beetroot can be slightly heating for Pitta, so enjoy this juice in moderation.
- Kapha: This juice is beneficial for Kapha due to its detoxifying and energizing effects.

Fenugreek Tea

A soothing and warming tea known for its potential to support healthy blood sugar levels.

Prep: 5 mins | Cook: 10 mins | Total: 10 mins | Serves: 1

Ingredients

- 1 teaspoon fenugreek seeds
- 1 cup filtered water

Ayurvedic Considerations

- Dosha: Balancing for all doshas, especially Vata
- Taste: Bitter
- Benefits: Supports healthy blood sugar levels, aids digestion, may help with lactation
- You can add a pinch of turmeric or ginger to enhance the flavor and health benefits.
- If the taste is too bitter, add a small amount of honey or jaggery.
- Drink this tea regularly to support your blood sugar balance

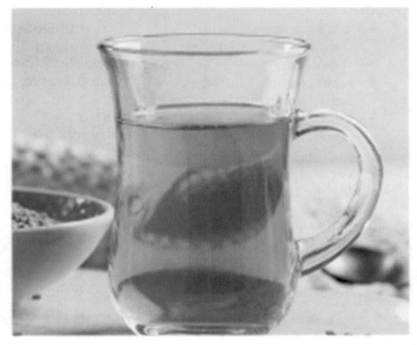

Preparation

1. Rinse the fenugreek seeds and place them in a small bowl or cup.
2. Pour the water over the seeds and let them soak overnight.
3. In the morning, transfer the soaked seeds and water to a small saucepan.
4. Heat until it starts to boil, then reduce heat and simmer for additional 10 minutes.
5. Strain the tea into a cup and discard the seeds.
6. Enjoy warm or let it cool.

Nutrition

Calories: 5 | Carbs: 1g | Protein: 0g | Fat: 0g

1. .

Aloe Vera Juice

A revitalizing and hydrating drink to soothe your system and promote inner balance. Aloe vera, revered in Ayurveda for its cooling and detoxifying properties, is combined with a hint of honey for natural sweetness and a touch of lime for a refreshing twist.

Prep: 5 mins | Total: 5 mins | Serves: 1

Ingredients

- 1/4 cup fresh aloe vera gel (sourced from the inner leaf of a mature aloe vera plant)
- 1 cup filtered water
- 1 teaspoon raw honey (optional)
- 1/4 lime, juiced (optional)

Ayurvedic Considerations

- Dosha Suitability: This drink is generally suitable for all doshas, but Pitta individuals may want to reduce or omit the honey to avoid excess heat.
- Benefits: Aloe vera is cooling, detoxifying, and hydrating, while honey is nourishing and soothing. Lime aids digestion.
- If fresh aloe vera is unavailable, you can use pure aloe vera juice, ensuring it's free from added sugars or preservatives

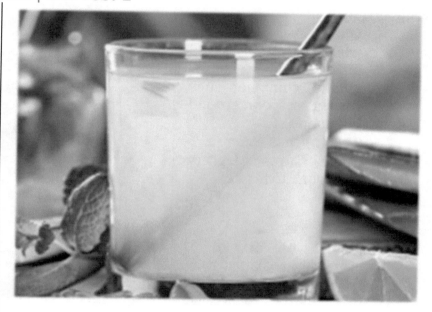

Preparation

2. Carefully extract the clear aloe vera gel from a mature leaf. Rinse the gel to remove any impurities.
3. Blend the aloe vera gel with filtered water until smooth.
4. Add honey and lime juice to taste.

Nutrition

Calories: 20 | Carbs: 5g | Sugar: 5g

Ginger and Cinnamon Tea

This warming and aromatic tea is a simple yet powerful Ayurvedic remedy for improving digestion and circulation. Ginger's pungent heat stimulates digestive fire (agni), while cinnamon's sweetness balances Vata dosha and supports blood sugar levels.

Prep: 5 mins | Cook: 10-12 mins | Total: 15-17 mins | Serves: 1

Ingredients

- One (1)-inch piece fresh, peeled and thinly sliced ginger root
- One (1) cinnamon stick (or 1/2 teaspoon ground cinnamon)
- Two (2) cups water
- Honey or jaggery (optional, to taste)

Ayurvedic Considerations

- This tea is balancing for all doshas, but particularly beneficial for Vata and Kapha due to its warming properties.
- For Pitta dosha, you can reduce the amount of ginger or omit it altogether.

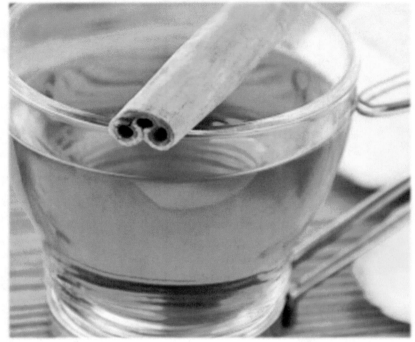

Preparation

1. In a small saucepan, combine the ginger slices, cinnamon stick, and water.
2. Heat the saucepan until it ton boil, then reduce heat and simmer for additional 10 mins.
3. Remove from heat and strain the tea into a mug.
4. Add the sweetener (honey or jaggery) to taste, if desired.

Nutrition

Calories: 10.5 | Carbs: 2g | Protein: 0g | Fat: 1g

Chapter

Conclusion

The journey through the pages of this Ayurvedic cookbook for women has been a flavorful exploration of ancient wisdom and modern nourishment. As you've discovered, Ayurveda offers a holistic approach to women's health, embracing not only the physical body but also the mind and spirit. By incorporating Ayurvedic principles into your kitchen and lifestyle, you've embarked on a path towards hormonal harmony, radiant well-being, and a deeper connection with your feminine essence.

The recipes within this book are more than just kitchen creations; they are tools for self-care and empowerment. Each dish has been carefully crafted to balance the doshas, nourish the body, and support hormonal health at every stage of a woman's life. From warming breakfasts to satisfying dinners, revitalizing drinks, and delectable desserts, these recipes offer a symphony of flavors that delight the senses while promoting optimal well-being.

Beyond the kitchen, the Ayurvedic rituals and practices shared in this book provide a roadmap for cultivating a balanced and fulfilling lifestyle. By incorporating daily routines, seasonal practices, stress management techniques, and mindful eating habits, you can create a harmonious rhythm that supports your body's natural cycles and fosters a deep sense of inner peace.

As you continue on your Ayurvedic journey, remember that true health is a lifelong pursuit. Embrace the wisdom of this ancient science, listen to your body's unique needs, and trust your intuition. By nourishing yourself with wholesome foods, practicing mindful movement, and cultivating a peaceful mind, you can unlock your full potential and radiate vibrant health from the inside out.

May this cookbook serve as a trusted companion on your path to optimal well-being. May it inspire you to embrace the rich flavors and healing traditions of Ayurveda, and may it empower you to create a life that is both nourishing and fulfilling. As you savor each bite and embrace each practice, may you experience the profound joy of living in harmony with your true nature as a woman.

BONUSES

DEAR READER

Your journey through the flavors and wisdom of Ayurveda has been a true inspiration to us. As you continue to explore the recipes and practices within these pages, we invite you to share your experience with us. Your feedback is invaluable in helping us create resources that truly nourish and empower women on their path to well-being.

We'd be delighted if you could take a moment to leave an honest review of this cookbook. Your insights, whether they be about a favorite recipe, a transformative ritual, or a newfound understanding of Ayurvedic principles, will help guide other women on their own journeys. By sharing your thoughts, you become a part of our growing community of women supporting and inspiring each other. We are deeply grateful for your support and look forward to hearing your voice.

30 Day Meal Planner

Day	Breakfast	Lunch	Dinner	Snacks
1	Warm Spiced Oatmeal	Kitchari	Baked Salmon with Lemon and Dill	Spiced Nuts and Seeds
2	Chickpea Flour Pancakes	Red Lentil Soup with Coconut Milk and Turmeric	Chicken Curry with Coconut Milk and Spinach	Fruit Salad with Mint and Lime
3	Coconut Milk Chia Seed Pudding	Roasted Vegetable Salad with Tahini Dressing	Vegetable Stir-Fry with Ginger and Garlic	Ayurvedic Date and Nut Energy Balls
4	Spiced Carrot and Ginger Muffins	Sweet Potato and Chickpea Curry	Cauliflower Rice with Turmeric and Peas	Avocado and Egg Toast
5	Golden Milk Smoothie	Spiced Lentil Wraps with Avocado and Greens	Sweet Potato and Black Bean Tacos	Ayurvedic Spiced Popcorn
6	Sweet Potato and Coconut Flour Pancakes	Vegetable Curry & Coconut Rice	Baked Chicken with Turmeric and Lemon	Apple Slices with Almond Butter
7	Ayurvedic Quinoa Bowl	Lentil and Spinach Soup with Lemon and Ginger	Ayurvedic Vegetable Biryani	Cucumber Raita

8	Spiced Apple and Pear Porridge	Quinoa Tabbouleh Salad	Salmon with Roasted Vegetables and Tahini Sauce	Hard-Boiled Eggs with Turmeric
9	Banana and Almond Butter Smoothie	Sweet Potato and Black Bean Burger	Roasted Vegetable Curry with Tofu or Tempeh	Spiced Carrot Sticks with Hummus
10	Spiced Carrot and Zucchini Bread	Lentil Vegetable Fritters with Yogurt Dip	One-Pan Lemon Herb Chicken and Vegetables	Baked Kale Chips
11	Oatmeal with Eggs and Greens	Roasted Vegetable Salad with Turmeric Tahini Dressing	Butternut Squash and Chickpea Curry with Spinach	Banana Nice Cream
12	Buckwheat Pancakes with Berries and Yogurt	Quinoa Black Bean Salad with Avocado Dressing	Baked Cod with Turmeric and Ginger	Guacamole with Veggie Sticks
13	Golden Milk Chia Seed Pudding	Chickpea Curry with Spinach and Coconut Milk	Sweet Potato Black Bean Enchiladas	Spiced Nuts and Seeds
14	Savory Mung Bean Pancakes	Spiced Lentil and Brown Rice Bowl	Creamy Coconut Lentil Curry	Fruit Salad with Mint and Lime
15	Sweet Potato Breakfast Bowl	Roasted Cauliflower and Chickpea Salad	Baked Salmon with Lemon and Dill	Ayurvedic Date and Nut Energy Balls

16	Spiced Coconut Milk Porridge	Sweet Potato and Lentil Curry with Coconut Milk	Chicken Curry with Coconut Milk and Spinach	Avocado and Egg Toast
17	Buckwheat and Berry Smoothie	Kitchari	Vegetable Stir-Fry with Ginger and Garlic	Ayurvedic Spiced Popcorn
18	Warm Spiced Oatmeal	Red Lentil Soup with Coconut Milk and Turmeric	Cauliflower Rice with Turmeric and Peas	Apple Slices with Almond Butter
19	Chickpea Flour Pancakes	Roasted Vegetable Salad with Tahini Dressing	Sweet Potato and Black Bean Tacos	Cucumber Raita
20	Coconut Milk Chia Seed Pudding	Sweet Potato and Chickpea Curry	Baked Chicken with Turmeric and Lemon	Hard-Boiled Eggs with Turmeric
21	Spiced Carrot and Ginger Muffins	Spiced Lentil Wraps with Avocado and Greens	Ayurvedic Vegetable Biryani	Spiced Carrot Sticks with Hummus
22	Golden Milk Smoothie	Vegetable Curry & Coconut Rice	Salmon with Roasted Vegetables and Tahini Sauce	Baked Kale Chips
23	Sweet Potato and Coconut Flour Pancakes	Lentil and Spinach Soup with Lemon and Ginger	Roasted Vegetable Curry with Tofu or Tempeh	Banana Nice Cream

24	Ayurvedic Quinoa Bowl	Quinoa Tabbouleh Salad	One-Pan Lemon Herb Chicken and Vegetables	Guacamole with Veggie Sticks
25	Spiced Apple and Pear Porridge	Sweet Potato and Black Bean Burger	Butternut Squash and Chickpea Curry with Spinach	Spiced Nuts and Seeds
26	Banana and Almond Butter Smoothie	Lentil Vegetable Fritters with Yogurt Dip	Baked Cod with Turmeric and Ginger	Fruit Salad with Mint and Lime
27	Spiced Carrot and Zucchini Bread	Roasted Vegetable Salad with Turmeric Tahini Dressing	Sweet Potato Black Bean Enchiladas	Ayurvedic Date and Nut Energy Balls
28	Oatmeal with Eggs and Greens	Quinoa Black Bean Salad with Avocado Dressing	Creamy Coconut Lentil Curry	Avocado and Egg Toast
29	Buckwheat Pancakes with Berries and Yogurt	Chickpea Curry with Spinach and Coconut Milk	Baked Salmon with Lemon and Dill	Ayurvedic Spiced Popcorn
30	Golden Milk Chia Seed Pudding	Spiced Lentil and Brown Rice Bowl	Chicken Curry with Coconut Milk and Spinach	Apple Slices with Almond Butter

INDEX

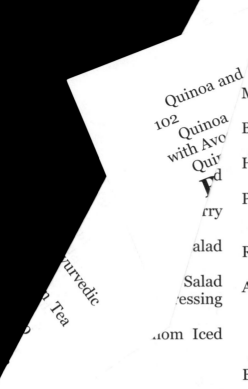

REFERENCE

CANVA.COM – All images used are attributed to Canva Pro

Made in United States
Troutdale, OR
09/29/2024